Pocket Medical Dictionary

In Association with the Royal Society
of Medicine

D0682706

Longman

Foreword

Compiled with the help of the Royal
Society of Medicine this book
contains those medical words which,
when used by a doctor, often mystify,
and may worry, the patient. The
definitions given here clearly and
simply explain body processes,
illnesses, and types of bugs and
drugs. As a further guide to those
alarming-sounding words, a short
supplementary glossary is provided
which gives the Latin and Greek roots
of much medical vocabulary.
Cross-references within the text are
indicated by SMALL CAPITALS.

A

The moving of a part away from its midline or from the axis of the body; for example, moving the arm away from the body. The opposite of ADDUCTION.	**Abduction**
Blood groups are based on the presence or absence of factors in red blood cells, determined by heredity. Type A blood contains factor A; type B blood contains factor B; type AB contains both factors; type O contains neither. These types are further subdivided by the presence or absence of anti-A or anti-B factors in red cells or serum, and by even more complicated factors.	**ABO**
Expulsion of an embryo or fetus from the uterus before it is capable of independent life. *Spontaneous* abortion is not uncommon; the lay term is miscarriage. Some expulsions of an embryo too malformed to live occur so early in pregnancy that they may not be recognized. *Induced* abortions, performed under safe and sterile conditions in a hospital, are permissible if doctors agree that the mother's life or health is endangered. *Criminal* abortions (illegal operations) are performed under conditions of furtiveness, crudity, and haste which can lead to infection, sterility, and even death.	**Abortion**
A scraped skin surface, such as a grazed knee which oozes blood.	**Abrasion**
A collection of pus within a well-defined space in any part of the body. Treatment is by drainage and overcoming the infection.	**Abscess**
Change in curvature of the lens of the eye to bring objects into sharp focus.	**Accommodation**
The French word for childbirth.	**Accouchement**
The cup-shaped cavity in the pelvis in which the upper end of the femur rests.	**Acetabulum**
Inability to relax a hollow muscular organ; especially, the lower portion of the oesophagus (*cardiospasm*), producing a	**Achalasia**

A

Achilles tendon	feeling that swallowed food has lodged itself at the entrance to the stomach.

The thickest and strongest tendon of the body, extending upwards about 15 cm from the back of the heel. It binds the muscles of the calf of the leg to the bone in the heel. |
Achlorhydria	Absence of free hydrochloric acid in the stomach. The condition is a feature of pernicious anaemia, sometimes of stomach cancer or other diseases, but it may occur in elderly people who are quite healthy.
Acholic	Without bile. Clay-coloured *acholic stools* indicate some obstructive disorder of the liver or bile ducts.
Achondroplasia	A form of dwarfism; the head and torso are of normal size but arms and legs are very short. The condition results from a congenital defect in the formation of cartilage at the growing ends of long bones which prevents normal lengthening.
Acid and alkaline foods	There is no reason for a normal person to be in the least concerned about the acidity or alkalinity of foods. Doctors sometimes put patients who have acid kidney stones on a high alkaline ash diet, and patients who have alkaline kidney stones on a high acid ash diet. Persons with peptic ulcer should not drink large amounts of citrus or other acid juices on an empty stomach, because the immediate effect is to increase acidity and irritate the ulcer. But the ultimate effect of most acid juices and of foods which contain organic acids and taste sour is to leave an alkaline ash – that is, their ultimate reactions in the body are alkaline. Almost all fruits and vegetables, although they may taste acid, are alkaline-producing foods. The major acid-producing foods are cereals, meats, eggs, and cheese, which do not taste acid at all. An odinary mixed diet provides perfectly adequate acid-alkaline ash balance, and even if it does not, the body has remarkably efficient buffering systems to maintain a balance. *Foods with alkaline ash* All fruits except cranberries, plums, prunes, and rhubarb All vegetables except maize and dried lentils Milk Almonds Brazil nuts Chestnuts Coconut Treacle *Foods with*

acid ash	Bread	Cereals	Cranberries, plums,
prunes, rhubarb	Bacon	Beef	Cheese	Chicken

acid ash   Bread   Cereals   Cranberries, plums, prunes, rhubarb   Bacon   Beef   Cheese   Chicken   Eggs   Fish   Ham   Lamb   Liver   Pork   Veal   Peanut butter   Peanuts   Walnuts   Maize   Lentils *Neutral foods*   Butter   Cornflour   Cream   Lard   Oils   Sugar   Tapioca   Coffee   Tea

Acid-base balance

Blood is slightly alkaline; it is never acid during life. Mechanisms which maintain this delicate balance are remarkably efficient and do not require attention except in presence of disease which a doctor can recognize. Acid-base balance is kept constant by elimination of carbon dioxide from the lungs, excretion of acid by the kidneys (urine is normally acid), and buffer systems of the blood. The chief acid-maker is carbon dioxide, which forms carbonic acid when dissolved in water. Sodium bicarbonate constitutes a large alkaline reserve in the blood. Interplay between carbonic acid and bicarbonate keeps the blood balanced. *Acidosis* (reduced alkalinity of the blood, but not to the extent that it becomes acid) can result from disturbance of the balancing system by kidney insufficiency, diabetes, prolonged diarrhoea with loss of bicarbonate, and other conditions. Significant acidosis practically never occurs except in diseases which are or should be under treatment. Strenuous exercise can also produce mild and harmless acidosis because breathing cannot quite keep pace with carbon dioxide accumulation. Excessive intake of antacids or bicarbonate may produce the opposite condition, *alkalosis*, slightly increased alkalinity of the blood. Alkalosis may be induced by hyperventilation; overbreathing washes out carbon dioxide. The same type of alkalosis occurs in MOUNTAIN SICKNESS when overbreathing results from thinness of the air at high altitudes. Alkalosis can result from prolonged vomiting which removes a large amount of acid from the system.

Acidosis

Decreased alkalinity of the blood and other body fluids. See ACID-BASE BALANCE.

Acid stomach

Burning, gnawing pain in the upper abdomen is often attributed by the layman to acid stomach, especially if distress is not continuous. The stomach is naturally acid. Stomach discomfort may be due to hunger, or inflation by gas-producing foods, or irritants, or too much smoking, or food allergy, or overeating, or a dozen causes other than acid. If distress persists, see a doctor; it is unwise to take antacids continuously over long periods to subdue symptoms when some possibly serious condition is involved.

Acne rosacea

A chronic disease, entirely unrelated to common acne, resulting from dilatation of superficial blood vessels, giving an appearance of constant redness to the area of the middle part of the face.

Acne vulgaris

Common acne; a skin disorder, most conspicuously affecting the face, with pimples and blackheads as the most obvious lesions. Acne has nothing to do with 'bad blood"; it is due to overactivity of oil-secreting glands and hair follicles. It is associated with the increase of sex hormones at puberty, and is in large degree a physiological condition that most young people pass through on their way to sexual maturity. Acne usually subsides in the twenties, but in the meantime various treatments are beneficial. Severe cases should have good medical care in order to prevent scarring and pitting.

Acromegaly

A disorder of adults due to overproduction of growth hormone by the pituitary gland. The word means 'large extremities." There is enlargement of the bones and soft parts of the face, hands, and feet. The face with its thickened tissues, enlarged jaw, nose, and bony ridges over the eyes, has a characteristic appearance. Height is not increased. However, if the same hormone overproduction occurs in a young person before the growing ends of the bones have closed, he becomes a giant up to eight feet tall (gigantism).

ACTH

Abbreviation of *adrenocorticotrophic hormone*; a hormone of the pituitary gland which stimulates the adrenal gland to produce cortisone.

Actinomycosis

(called by farmers 'wooden tongue") An infectious disease caused by fungi which produce unsightly lumpy pus-draining abscesses, especially common on the face and jaw.

The degree of sharpness of sight or hearing.	**Acuity**

An ancient Oriental (especially Chinese) system of folk medicine in which needles are inserted into parts of the body and twisted, to treat disease or induce anaesthesia. Traditional acupuncture recognizes about 300 regions of the body arranged on lines associated with major organs. Theoretically, needles inserted into appropriate sites on appropriate lines restore the ebb and flow of opposing forces (*yin* and *yang*; male and female) to natural rhythms, thus benefiting affected organs. Interest of Western physicians in the theories and mysteries of acupuncture was stimulated by doctors who visited China and watched major operations in which acupuncture was apparently used successfully as the only form of anaesthesia. A few experiments with acupuncture (modified, in some instances, by attaching a source of electric current to needles instead of (twisting them) suggest that the procedure might have limited value for anaesthesia in some circumstances. Whether acupuncture is a temporary fad, how many of its anaesthetizing effects are attributable to autohypnosis, and whether it is really practical, are undetermined. Hypnosis itself can produce anaesthesia, but few doctors use it because of time required for preparation and induction, and alternatives are always at hand, as with acupuncture. A disadvantage of acupuncture in major surgery is that, while it may ease pain, it does not – unlike conventional anaesthetics – produce muscle relaxation, which is important in surgical procedures.

Acupuncture

A chronic disease characterized by weakness, easy fatigability, skin pigmentation, low blood pressure, and other symptoms. The underlying cause is atrophy or disease of the outer layer of the adrenal gland.

Addison's disease

The moving of a part towards another or towards the axis of the body: for example, moving the thumb towards the index finger. The opposite of ABDUCTION.

Adduction

Adenoviruses

A group of viruses responsible for respiratory infections like the common cold, viral conjunctivitis, intestinal infections, and intestinal infections which may cause swelling of tonsils, adenoids, and other glandular tissue, especially in children. There are more than 30 different types of adenoviruses. They are widespread and sometimes give rise to epidemics. Most people have been infected by them. Except in small infants, adenovirus infections are rarely serious. They generally run their course in a week or less. Vaccines have been developed but their use is largely limited to military establishments where conditions are favourable for epidemics among young people.

Adhesions

Abnormal sticking together of tissues which should slip or slide freely over each other. Diseases may produce adhesions: in the chest cavity as a result of pleurisy, in injured joints restricted in movement, and in other areas of inflammation. Adhesions in the abdominal and pelvic cavities may occur after surgical operations, particulary if pus has spilled from a ruptured abscess. It is not usually desirable to perform further surgery to free the adhesions unless they threaten to obstruct the bowel.

Adipose tissue

Fatty connective tissue; commonly, the part of the body where fat is stored. Usually, adiposity is a way of saying 'too fat'.

Adiposis dolorosa

See DERCUM'S DISEASE.

Adolescence

The years between the beginning of puberty, when the reproductive organs become functionally active, and maturity.

Adolescent bent hip

A condition of older children resulting from disconnection of the upper end of the thighbone from its normal hip joint attachments, producing a wobbly painful hip, and limping.

Adrenalin

The hormone produced by the medulla of the adrenal gland. It stimulates heart action, constricts blood vessels, relaxes small bronchial tubes and other smooth muscle, and has many medical uses in allergic and other disorders. Also known as epinephrine.

Usually describes bacteria which live or function in air or free oxygen.	**Aerobic**
The study of causes of disease or disorder. Aetiology is not a word which means causes, but rather the study of causes.	**Aetiology**
A disease with a high fatality rate caused by organisms that get into the blood through the bites of tsetse flies indigenous to parts of Africa. It is not the same as sleepiness associated with some forms of encephalitis.	**African sleeping sickness**
The placenta and membranes discharged from the uterus a few minutes after the birth of a baby.	**Afterbirth**
A visual image which remains for a few seconds after the eyes are closed or light has ceased to stimulate. An after-image can be produced by looking at a bright light or bright objects for a few seconds, then closing the eyes, or turning them on a dark surface, or fixing the gaze on a bright sheet of white paper. An image of the object will slowly float into view, become more distinct, and gradually fade away. After-images are either positive or negative. A positive after-image shows the object in its correct shade of black or white or colour. A negative after-image reverses dark and light parts and, if the object was coloured, shows the complementary instead of the original colour; for instance, a red object produces a green after-image. NEVER LOOK DIRECTLY AT THE SUN.	**After-image**
Blood deficiency of GAMMA GLOBULIN, protein molecules which produce protective antibodies against infections. The deficiency leaves the patient extremely susceptible to infections.	**Agammaglobulinaemia**
An acute, rare, and sometimes fatal illness associated with extreme reduction or complete absence of granular white blood cells from the bone marrow and blood. Absence of cells which protect against infection results in weakness, rapid onset of fever, sore throat, prostration, ulceration of the mouth and mucous membranes. The disease may arise from unknown causes, but usually it can be traced to some chemical or drug	**Agranulocytosis**

which injures the bone marrow; the agent may be a widely used valuable drug which is harmless to most people but to which the patient is peculiarly sensitive. Treatment aims to combat infection while the bone marrow becomes normal.

Air embolism

Plugging of blood vessels by air bubbles carried in the bloodstream, fatal if large numbers of bubbles reach the heart. Air can enter the bloodstream by accidental injection or through wounds of the neck. Air embolism is also a hazard of scuba diving; holding the breath while ascending from even relatively shallow depths may cause rupture of a part of the lung, forcing air bubbles into the pulmonary veins and thence to arteries of the brain.

Air-swallowing
(*aerophagy*)

The habit, usually unconscious, of swallowing excessive amounts of air. The gas may escape by a belch, or lead to FLATULENCE, or may cause distension of the gut. A small amount of air is naturally swallowed with food or drink or conversation, but excessive intake may be promoted by gulping, chewing with the lips parted, drinking fluids from a narrow-necked bottle, talking while eating, chewing gum, smoking, and nervous swallowing. More often than not the air-swallower has no idea that he is doing it, and is usually able to overcome the habit if it is called to his attention.

Albumin

One of the proteins in blood plasma.

Albuminuria

Presence in the urine of albumin, a protein like egg white. The kidneys do not normally excrete albumin, which is a useful substance, and albuminuria suggests damage to the filtering apparatus, but this is not always the case.

Aldosteronism (primary)

A remediable form of high blood pressure with weakness, headaches, and other symptoms, due to excessive production of aldosterone, a hormone produced by the cortex of the adrenal gland. The hormone is a powerful regulator of salt and water balance. Excess causes retention of sodium and loss of potassium. If the excess is caused by an adrenal gland tumour, its removal is indicated. All the manifestations of primary aldosteronism can be reversed in a few weeks by oral doses of an antagonistic drug, spironolactone.

A diet consisting mainly of fruits and vegetables, with only small amounts of meat and cereals, sometimes prescribed for patients who have kidney disease or kidney stones of the uric acid type. Alkaline environment has been found to deter the formation of acid stones.	**Alkaline ash diet**
Increased alkalinity of the blood. See ACID-BASE BALANCE.	**Alkalosis**
A rare hereditary disorder in which the body is unable to produce enzymes for the proper utilization of certain AMINO ACIDS of protein foods. By-products of incomplete metabolism cause the urine to turn dark brown on long standing. The disorder does not affect life expectancy but in later life leads to discoloration of cartilage and possibly to a severe form of arthritis.	**Alkaptonuria**
A substance that produces ALLERGY.	**Allergen**
A capacity to react abnormally to specific substances which cause no symptoms in most people; a general term for all kinds of hypersensitivities. Atopy is a synonym for allergy.	**Allergy**
A drug which reduces the body's production of uric acid; used in treatment of GOUT.	**Allopurinol**
	Alopecia

Baldness; loss of head hair. Some types of hair loss are temporary, some are irreversible. Neither hair tonics nor any other medical measure can overcome male pattern baldness. This type affects men who have a genetic predisposition, who produce adequate amounts of male hormone, and who have attained puberty. New surgical techniques for transplanting hairs from an area of growth to the bare scalp have some success but are not widely popular. The technique consists of punching plugs of skin containing four or five hairs out of the back of the neck and inserting them into the scalp in hope that they will take root and spread. In time, after transplants of scores of tufts, the plugs may grow together to cover the scalp.

Alveolus   A sac or chamber; a saclike dilatation at the end of a passage; especially, an air cell of the lung, the bony socket of a tooth, or certain cells of the stomach.

Amblyopia   Dimness of vision without any organic lesion of the eye. Amblyopia may result from various toxins, or an eye, such as a squinting eye, may lose its vision from long disuse.

Amenorrhoea   The abnormal absence of menstruation.

Amino acids   Building blocks of PROTEIN. There are about twenty important amino acids. An amino acid molecule has an acid group of atoms at one end and an amino (nitrogen-containing) group at the other. In between are carbon units with different side chains which give each amino acid its individuality. The acid end of an amino acid links with the amino end of another, a sort of chemical hook-and-eye arrangement. In this way amino acids form short chains (peptides) or large complex molecules containing many hundreds of different amino acids in exact sequences (protein). Eight amino acids are called essential because the body cannot synthesize them and they must be obtained ready-made from protein foods. The amino acids of protein foods are separated by digestion and go into a general pool from which the body takes the ones it needs to synthesize its own proteins; thus an amino acid which we may have obtained from a pork chop may become a part of a fingernail, skin, hair, of a hormone such as insulin, or of an enzyme that activates some vital chemical process.

Amnion   The innermost of the fetal membranes, forming the BAG OF WATERS which surrounds and protects the developing child.

Amoebiasis   Amoebic dysentery.

Amyloidosis   Abnormal masses of protein infiltrating various organs; primary or secondary to chronic diseases; treatment depends on the underlying disease. Diagnosed by biopsy.

Amyotonia   Lack of muscle tone; a congenital form in infants is characterized by small underdeveloped muscles and weakness of the limbs and trunk.

A disease of the spinal cord which produces progressive paralysis and wasting of muscles on both sides of the body.	**Amyotrophic lateral sclerosis**
Drugs related to male hormones, sometimes given for anabolic (building-up) action, to stimulate growth, weight gain, strength, and appetite. The drugs are more accurately called androgenic-anabolic steriods, since they are related to testosterone and retain some of the male hormone's masculinizing action. Although the masculinizing action has been minimized in some anabolic steriods, the separation is not complete and prolonged use in women or children will cause virilization.	**Anabolic steroids**
The building-up part of metabolism; constructive processes of body cells which build complex substances from simpler ones. The opposite of CATABOLISM.	**Anabolism**
Usually describes bacteria which live or function in the absence of free air or free oxygen. TETANUS and GAS GANGRENE organisms are anaerobic. Such organisms thrive best where there is no oxygen, as in deep puncture wounds, and cannot survive if oxygen is present.	**Anaerobic**
Loss of feeling. This can occur from natural processes or accidents; for example, nerve injury, frostbite, hysteria, blood vessel spasms, etc. Ordinarily the word refers to obliteration of pain by anaesthetic drugs, with or without loss of consciousness. There are many kinds of anaesthetic drugs and gases, administered by inhalation, infusion, or injection. Each anaesthetic has specific properties, advantages, and disadvantages; selection of the best agent or combination for a particular patient requires special knowledge. The safety and relative comfort of modern surgery, and the ability to perform complex prolonged operations without haste, depend upon the anaesthesia team.	**Anaesthesia**
Anaphylaxis is an ANTIGEN-ANTIBODY reaction which occurs in seconds or minutes after a foreign substance has entered the body. The immediate, severe, and sometimes fatal reaction is	**Anaphylaxis**

manifested by nettle rash (urticaria), rhinitis, wheezing, shock, ANGIONEUROTIC OEDEMA, and difficult breathing, in varying combinations and degrees of severity. The most frequent causes of anaphylactic reactions are sera, drugs, and vaccines; next most common are insect stings. Skin tests may detect hypersensitivity to a substance, but sometimes even the minute amount used in a test may provoke a reaction. If a doctor asks you to wait for fifteen minutes or so after giving an injection, it is not a waste of time; he has emergency measures at hand if a dangerous reaction occurs. Because accident victims are often given routine injections of tetanus antitoxin or penicillin, persons who know they are sensitive to these substances should carry a warning card in their wallet or handbag where a doctor who is a stranger is sure to see it.

Anasarca	Generalized OEDEMA.
Androgen	A substance which has masculinizing effects.
Aneurysm	A blood-filled sac formed by dilatation of artery walls; it is susceptible to rupture and haemorrhage.
Angiitis	Inflammation of a blood or lymph vessel.
Angina pectoris	A crushing or gripping pain in the chest, often related to exertion or excitement, caused by insufficient blood passing through the coronary arteries of the heart.
Angiogram	An X-ray of blood vessels, usually performed by injecting a substance which is opaque to X-rays into the bloodstream. X-ray films in rapid succession may give important information about blood vessels in some types of heart trouble.
Angioma	A tumour composed of blood vessels; one kind of birthmark.
Angioneurotic oedema	Acute local swelling, like giant nettle rash under the skin, frequently a result of food allergy. The swelling is serious if it occurs around the tongue and larynx, threatening suffocation.

A

Abnormal deficiency of sweat production.	**Anhidrosis**
Stiffening or growing together of a joint; the fusion may be part of a disease process, or it may be a deliberate surgical immobilization.	**Ankylosis**
Deviation from normal of an organ or part; abnormality of structure or location.	**Anomaly**
Loss of appetite.	**Anorexia**
A nervous disorder manifested by profound aversion from food, leading to extreme emaciation. The typical patient is a young single woman. Usually she is not particularly concerned about her extreme thiness and may even insist that she eats a lot. Management of the condition requires explanation, encouragement of eating, possibly hospitalization and psychiatric help.	**Anorexia nervosa**
Deficiency of oxygen in the blood.	**Anoxaemia**
Oxygen deficiency in organs and tissues and the disturbance resulting therefrom.	**Anoxia**
A substance that counteracts or neutralizes acidity. Most commonly, a substance taken to reduce the acidity of gastric juice.	**Antacid**
A bacterial disease of herbivorous animals. The causal organism sometimes infects persons who have close contact with raw wool, bristles, or hides.	**Anthrax** (*wool-sorter's disease*)
Chemical substances produced by certain living cells, such as bacteria, yeasts, and moulds, that are antagonistic or damaging to certain other living cells, such as disease-producing bacteria. Different antibiotics may kill disease germs or prevent them from growing and multiplying.	**Antibiotics**
A protein in the blood, modified by contact with a foreign substance (*antigen*) so that it exerts an antagonizing or neutra-	**Antibody**

lizing action against that specific substance. Antibodies are chiefly associated with GAMMA GLOBULIN in the blood and are key elements of IMMUNITY mechanisms of the body. Usually the antibody-antigen reaction is protective. Measles virus is an antigen which stimulates the body to produce measles antibodies, so measles seldom occurs twice. But antibody-antigen reactions may also be distressing or harmful, as in allergies. So-called AUTO-IMMUNE DISEASES presumably result, at least in part, from harmful reactions of antibodies against normal proteins of the patient's own body.

Anticoagulants	Drugs which slow down the clotting process of the blood. Clots forming in blood vessels are potentially dangerous (see THROMBOSIS, EMBOLISM). Anticoagulants are useful in reducing the clotting tendency. The doctor's problem is knowing when and when not to use them; administration requires frequent checks of the patient's blood since overdosage can induce haemorrhage. Anticoagulants are sometimes given to patients for a few weeks after a heart attack caused by a blood clot in coronary arteries. There is wide difference of medical opinion as to whether the drugs should be continued for preventitive purposes for many months or years or the remainder of a lifetime.
Anticonvulsants	Drugs which are used to reduce the number and severity of chronic epileptic seizures. The doctor's choice of drugs depends upon the type of seizure. Since the drugs must be used for a prolonged period, it is important that the patient be told of possible adverse effects and be instructed to report unusual symptoms to his doctor.
Antidiuretic hormone	A hormone produced in brain areas linked with the pituitary gland; it checks the secretion of urine.
Antiemetic	A drug or treatment which stops or prevents nausea or vomiting.
Antigen	Any substance which stimulates the production of ANTIBODIES.

A large family of drugs which block some of the effects of histamine, a normal substance in body cells which play a part in allergic reactions. Histamine, triggered by an allergen, may escape from local groups of cells and cause symptoms of hay fever. Deliberate injection of histamine causes the walls of capillaries to become so permeable that fluids leak into nearby tissues. This leakage is characteristic of allergies. The effect may be superficial, as in weepy eyes or running nose or nettle rash, or more deep-set, as in dangerous swelling and constriction of the breathing passages. Antihistamine drugs are most effective in the treatment of acute nettle rash and seasonal hay fever, and generally give good results in subduing allergic tissue swellings (angioneurotic oedema). They may often give symptomatic relief of allergic skin disorders and of itching which is not of allergic origin. The most widely prescribed preventitives for motion sickness belong to the antihistamine family; they are effective against symptoms of dizziness, nausea, and vomiting, and have some sedative action. Although many attacks of asthma are allergic in origin, antihistamines have only limited value in this disease. The drugs differ one from another in potency, effects, and duration of action; facts weighed by the doctor in prescribing a specific drug. Some antihistamines have a pronounced tendency to cause drowsiness; others have very little sedative action. A person taking an antihistamine with sedative action should be aware of its effects on driving ability. Some sleeping pills and insomnia remedies contain small amounts of an antihistamine compound. These may cause drowsiness but the effect is not uniform. Most persons will acquire tolerance to the drug, and antihistamines cannot be considered reliable remedies against insomnia. Because of the depressant action of antihistamines, patients should not drink alcoholic beverages or take barbiturates which in combination may magnify depressant effects.

Prevention of ERYTHROBLASTOSIS (Rh disease) is now possible. Pregnant women lacking a substance in their red blood cells (Rh factor) may develop ANTIBODIES against their own babies whose blood does possess the factor. These antibodies can cause severe anaemia and damage to the unborn child. The risk increases with each pregnancy after the first, which usually is normal because the mother has not yet become sensitized. A preventitive measure is treatment of the Rh-negative mother with a specially prepared anti-Rh serum after the birth of each Rh-positive baby, to destroy quickly any Rh-positive blood cells of the baby which might have entered her circulation, thus greatly reducing the chance of her sensitization. Wide use of the serum may in the future eliminate this important cause of stillbirth and serious birth defects.

Antitoxin

A substance which neutralizes a specific bacterial, animal, or plant toxin. Most of the antitoxins injected by doctors for treatment or prevention of disease are prepared from serum obtained from a horse which has been immunized by gradually increased doses of a particular toxin. Harmful reactions may follow injection if a patient is sensitive to the serum component.

Antivenin

An antitoxin to venom, especially snake venom.

Antrum

See MAXILLARY SINUS.

Anuria

Total suppression of urine secretion; suggestive of but not confined to kidney damage.

Aorta

The great blood vessel which arches from the top of the heart and passes down through the chest and abdomen. It is the main trunk of the arterial system.

Aphakia

Absence of the lens of the eye, as after cataract surgery.

Aplastic anaemia

A grave form of anaemia due to progressive failure of the bone marrow to develop new blood cells; it may be caused by chemicals which poison the cell-producing mechanisms of the marrow.

Apnoea

Temporary cessation of breathing because of absence of stimulation of the breathing centre, as by too little carbon dioxide or too much oxygen.

Apoplexy

A stroke; cerebrovascular accident; rupture or haemorrhage of blood vessels in the brain.

Acute inflammation of the appendix. It occurs in all age groups but is most common in children and young persons. Typically, pain is felt in the region of the navel before it moves down to the appendix area in the lower right quarter of the abdomen, but not all cases are typical. The early pain may be mistaken for colic. If a child's severe stomachache persists for more than an hour or two, a doctor should be called to diagnose the trouble, which most often is not appendicitis, but if it is, prompt action is important because an inflamed appendix can reach bursting point in a few hours.	**Appendicitis**
These are drugs used to allay hunger and to make the early phases of adjusting to a diet easier. The drugs should be used only for a short time as adjuncts to a low-calorie diet for overcoming obesity, because long-continued use is habit-forming and dangerous.	**Appetite depressants** (*anorectic drugs*)
Watery fluid which fills the chamber of the eye in front of the lens. Obstruction of drainage causes pressures that lead to glaucoma.	**Aqueous humour**
A white ring around the outer edge of the cornea of the eye, especially in the aged.	**Arcus senilis**
A pigmented ring surrounding a central point; for example, the pigmented area encircling the nipple.	**Areola**
A pupil of the eye which does not react to light but does react to accommodation; a feature of syphilis of the central nervous system.	**Argyll Robertson pupil**
Any departure from normal rhythm of the heartbeat.	**Arrhythmia**
A thickening and hardening of the walls of arteries, leading to loss of their elasticity.	**Arteriosclerosis**
Mechanical introduction of semen into the vagina or uterus to induce pregnancy. If successful, conception, pregnancy, and	**Artificial insemination**

childbirth occur in a normal way. The first recorded attempt at human artificial insemination was performed by the famous surgeon, John Hunter, in 1799. Artificial insemination is widely employed in animal husbandry, but its availability to couples troubled by *infertility* has largely come about in the past twenty-five years. Technically, there are two forms of artificial insemination: AIH, in which semen is provided by the husband, and AID, in which semen is provided by a donor. Because the husband's infertility is usually the dominant factor, AID is the most frequently used method. There are no exact figures on the number of children conceived by artificial insemination, but the number runs into the thousands and some of these children have themselves become parents.

Artificial kidney

A device, of which there are several types, which passes a patient's blood over a membrane outside the body, to extract waste materials and return cleaned blood to the circulation.

Artificial pneumothorax

Surgical collapse of a lung for therapeutic purposes. Not much used now.

Asbestosis

Slowly progressing inflammation of the lungs, resulting from inhalation of fine asbestos fibres. It occurs in miners and workers in construction trades exposed to asbestos-containing materials. The lungs cannot eliminate asbestos dusts, and normal tissue is replaced by fibrous tissue; the incidence of a particular kind of cancer in persons with asbestosis is high.

Ascariasis

Infestation with a species of round-worms which inhabit the small bowel.

Ascites

Painless accumulation of yellowish fluid in the abdominal cavity, indicative of impaired circulation often related to heart failure, cirrhosis of the liver, malignancy, or kidney disease. Diuretic drugs or sodium and fluid restriction may control this, depending on the underlying disease.

Aspiration

Removal of fluids or gases from a body cavity by suction. Also, inhalation of foreign material, as in aspiration pneumonia.

A form of pneumonia caused by foreign matter in the lungs. The foreign substance may be inhaled, it may trickle into the windpipe, or it may be forced into the windpipe by choking or difficulties of swallowing. Lipoid or oil pneumonia can occur in infants and elderly persons. It is important to avoid putting oils into an infant's nose. Give oily substances such as cod liver oil only when the child is in an upright position and can swallow properly.	**Aspiration pneumonia**
A condition of paroxysmal, difficult, laboured, wheezy breathing.	**Asthma**
Distortion of vision resulting from imperfect curvature of the cornea or lens of the eye. The defect may be so slight that nothing need be done about it, or severe enough to cause eye strain. The condition is corrected by using a lens that bends light in only one direction.	**Astigmatism**
The anklebone	**Astragalus**
Loss of muscular coordination. There are many causes.	**Ataxia**
A retracted or collapsed state of the lung which leaves all or part of the organ airless. The condition may arise from obstruction of bronchial tubes; gases in the affected part of the lung are gradually absorbed and the area collapses. *Fetal atelectasis* is a condition in which the lungs of an infant do not expand adequately immediately after birth, as they normally should.	**Atelectasis**
A condition usually occurring in children as the result of a brain lesion, characterized by rhythmical movements of fingers, toes, or other parts.	**Athetosis**
See ALLERGY.	**Atopy**
Closure or failure to develop of a normal opening or channel in the body.	**Atresia**
Of or relating to the atria of the heart.	**Atrial**

Atrophy	Wasting away or shrinking in size of organ, tissue, or part.
Atypical pneumonia	See PNEUMONIA
Audiometer	An electrical instrument which emits pure tones that can be made louder or fainter. It is used in measuring acuity of hearing for sounds of different frequencies.
Aura	A premonitory sensation preceding an epileptic seizure.
Auscultation	Determination of the condition of organs, particularly the heart and lungs, by study of sounds arising from them.
Autoclave	An apparatus for sterilizing instruments by steam under pressure.
Autograft	A piece of tissue taken from one part of a patient's body and transplanted to another part, as in skin grafts to cover raw areas, burns, and so on.
Auto-immune diseases	Several diseases of unknown cause may reflect a strange inability of the body to 'recognize" itself, so that mechanisms which normally create immunity to foreign invaders establish a specific sensitivity to certain of the body's own tissues, with harmful consequences. The concept is complex, relatively new, and the mechanisms are not fully understood.
Avascular	Without blood or lymphatic vessels; the nails, the cornea, and some types of cartilage are avascular.
Avulsion	The forcible tearing away of a part.
Axilla	The armpit.
Axon	A single long fine fibre which conducts impulses away from the body of a nerve cell. Most axons are covered with a sheath of material called *myelin*; abnormalities of this covering occur in demyelinating diseases such as multiple sclerosis.
Azoospermia	Absence of active spermatozoa in semen.

B

Acute diarrhoea, acquired by person-to-person contact, eating contaminated objects, or through spread of contamination by flies. The causative germs are present in the excretions of infected persons. Infection is caused by rod-shaped bacteria called shigella, of which there are several types of variable virulence. Good sanitary and hygienic practices prevent infection. In infants and small children, bacillary dysentry can cause serious loss of fluids and ELECTROLYTES in a short time; the onset of severe diarrhoea is cause for calling a doctor promptly.

Bacillary dysentry (*shigellosis*)

The presence of living bacteria in circulating blood.

Bacteraemia

Tiny single-celled organisms. Bacteria can be seen with a microscope. They are shaped like spheres, rods, spirals, or commas. Most bacteria are harmless and even useful to man. Those which cause diseases are called *pathogenic* bacteria.

Bacteria

Chronic inflammation of the lungs caused by inhalation of bagasse, the material left from crushed sugar cane after its juices have been extracted.

Bagassosis

The fluid-filled sac which protects the fetus during pregnancy. During labour the bag of waters helps to dilate the outlet of the uterus for passage of the baby through the birth canal. Usually the bag of waters ruptures at the height of a strong contraction and the fluid escapes with a gush, but rupture may occur even before labour pains begin (dry labour).

Bag of waters

See ALOPECIA.

Baldness

An instrument for measuring the jerk given by the heartbeat to the body. It is useful in some aspects of diagnosis.

Ballistocardiograph

A spine deformed by ankylosing spondylitis, having the jointed appearance of bamboo.

Bamboo spine

Enlarged spleen and anaemia, associated with cirrhosis of the liver and ASCITES.

Banti's syndrome

Barber's itch
(*tinea sycosis*)

A fungus infection of bearded parts of the face, producing reddish patches covered with dry hairs or scales. A more severe condition, *sycosis barbae*, is caused by bacterial infecton of follicles of the beard, producing crusts, pimples, and numerous pustules perforated by hairs.

Barbiturates

Drugs now used mainly for the control of epilepsy. They have been superseded by safer drugs as sleeping pills. In the United Kingdom barbiturates have become much less popular with doctors in recent years, because they are habit-forming, they have bad long-term effects, they are liable to serious abuse by drug-takers, and used often to be taken for attempted suicide. A number of nonbarbiturate sleeping pills with a greater margin of safety than the barbiturates have been developed. All these drugs are sold only on medical prescription.

Barium meal and barium enema

A suspension of insoluble barium sulphate in water, swallowed in preparation for a stomach X-ray. The barium has greater density to X-rays than surrounding tissues and thus defines structures. To outline the large intestine the barium is given by enema.

Barrel chest

A rounded, bulging, barrel-shaped chest which moves poorly with the intake and output of air and is more or less fixed in a position of deep inhalation; characteristic of advanced emphysema.

Bartholin glands

Small glands on the floor and sides of the vaginal opening which secrete lubricating material. The glands are subject to infection and cyst formation.

Basal ganglia

Aggregations of nerve cells in the region of the base of the brain; Parkinson's disease is associated with abnormalities in this area.

Basal metabolic rate
(BMR)

A baseline of the minimal rate of energy expenditure for maintaining basal activities such as heart action, breathing, and heat production when the body is at rest; useful in diagnosis of certain diseases, especially those involving the thyroid gland.

B

Bacillus of Calmette and Guérin; a vaccine which gives immunity to tuberculosis for a variable time. The vaccine contains strains of live tubercle bacilli grown on ox bile for a long period to reduce their virulence. It is a safe vaccine, extensively used, mostly in persons with special hazards of exposure to tuberculosis, such as doctors, nurses, and members of families of tuberculosis patients. BCG vaccination interferes with the interpretation of tuberculin tests, but proponents point out that there are other ways of detecting tuberculous infection.	**BCG**
Twice a day.	**BDS**
Pains which occur in the second stage of labour when the mother, feeling that something must be expelled, makes powerful contractions of her abdominal muscles in coordination with the contractions of the uterus.	**Bearing down pains**
A frame to prevent the weight of bedclothing from pressing on a patient's body.	**Bed cradle**
PRESSURE SORES.	**Bedsores**
Nocturnal enuresis.	**Bed-wetting**
A nonvenereal form of syphilis, transmitted by such means as contaminated eating and drinking utensils. Occurs chiefly in the Middle East.	**Bejel**
Paralysis of the facial nerve, usually temporary; the patient is unable to move muscles of the mouth, eye, and forehead on one side.	**Bell's palsy**
An abnormal protein in the urine, occurring most often in association with *multiple myeloma*. The substance is readily deposited in the kidney tubules and leads to impaired kidney function.	**Bence Jones protein**
See CAISSON DISEASE.	**Bends**

Benign	Mild; usually the word means that a tumour is not cancerous. Benign tumours are not necessarily harmless; they can cause a wide range of symptoms related to pressure, obstruction, twisting, and excessive production of potent substances such as hormones.
Beriberi	A deficiency disease, rare in this country, chiefly the result of a deficiency of thiamine (vitamin B₁) in the diet. *Dry* beriberi chiefly affects the nerves of the extremities; *wet* beriberi is characterized by oedema and congestive heart failure.
Bezoar	A solid mass of compacted indigestible material in the stomach or intestines, found occasionally in mentally disturbed persons who swallow rags, hair, rope, and other inedible materials. A hair ball is called a *trichobezoar*.
Bile	A yellowish or greenish fluid continuously manufactured in the liver; it is stored and concentrated in the gallbladder and released as required into the duodenum. Bile helps to emulsify and absorb fats and to alkalinize the intestine. It is a complex, bitter-tasting fluid (gall) containing pigments, salts, fatty acids, cholesterol, and other materials. Bile salts are sometimes used in medicine to stimulate the secretory activity of the liver.
Bilharziasis	See SCHISTOSOMIASIS.
Biliousness	A nondescript word for vague symptoms attributed, usually wrongly, to the liver. Probably the word survives from ancient times when a 'choleric' person was said to have an excess of yellow bile and a 'melancholy' person an excess of black bile. Many symptoms, including jaundice, can indeed arise from abnormalities of bile, but only a doctor can diagnose them.
Bilirubin	The principal pigment of bile; a substance derived from the breakdown of HAEMOGLOBIN. Bilirubin tests are useful in determining the nature of certain blood and liver diseases, in distinguishing different types of jaundice, and in evaluating excessive destruction of blood cells.
Biological clocks	Some people can set a mental clock to awaken them before an

alarm clock goes off. A few are confident enough to dispense with alarm clocks entirely. Many familiar physiological rhythms recur approximately every 24 hours — sleep, waking, ups and downs of body temperature and heart rate. These are called *circadian rhythms*. There are also many shorter rhythms, such as brain wave patterns, superimposed upon longer ones. All of these are rather like biological clocks distributed through the body.

Biopsy

Removal of tissue from the living body for purposes of diagnosis, as in cases of suspected cancer. The specimen may be subjected to biochemical tests; more often, it is set in a paraffin block, cut into very thin slices, stained, and studied under a microscope. If necessary, the procedure can be completed in a few minutes by quick-freezing the tissue. This is frequently done while the patient remains under anaesthesia on the operating table and surgeons await the pathologist's verdict as to whether a tumour of the breast or other organ is or is not malignant.

Birth control

See CONTRACEPTION.

Birth defects

Some live newborn infants have abnormalities recognizable at birth. Some defects such as a slightly twisted toe or a cleft lip are obvious *congenital malformations* (present at birth). Others have abnormalities which are not recognizable at birth, but which become apparent as they grow older. Many abnormalities are relatively minor, and about 80 per cent of birth defects, including the most serious forms such as congenital malformations of the heart, can be corrected and treated. *Causes*, if not the total mechanisms, of some birth defects are known. Some are hereditary, determined by parental CHROMOSOMES, and genetic counselling is helpful to prospective parents concerned about some real or imagined abnormality that runs in the family (see MEDICAL GENETICS). Some defects are *environmental*, quite unrelated to heredity. A disturbance of the environment of the fetus may distort its growth. The best-known examples of environment-caused abnormalities is infection of the mother with German measles at a critical time of pregnancy. Some abnormalities are believed to be caused by a combination of hereditary and environmental factors, or by an accident at the time of delivery, as in cases of brain damage due to interruption of the oxygen supply to the newborn during delivery. *Time of vulnerability.* It is now well established that certain birth defects originate at a critical time of pregnancy; in general, during the first three months, at the time when the cells of the embryo are developing into arms and legs and vital organs. At this time the embryo is peculiarly vulnerable to harmful agents. Before then it is too young; afterwards, too old to be seriously affected. It has also been established that in early pregnancy, excessive amounts of alcohol and tobacco have similar harmful effects on the embryo.

Blackwater fever	An acute complication of MALARIA, especially in persons who have been treated with quinine. An attack is marked by high fever, shivering, and profound anaemia; the urine is very dark, hence the name.
Black widow spider (*Latrodectus mactans*)	A small black spider with a globe-shaped abdomen marked by a reddish design like an hourglass or dumbbell. Its bite is very painful and can be serious if treatment is neglected. This spider is not native to Britain, but is occasionally imported in crates of fruit.
Blastomycosis	A group of diseases caused by yeastlike fungi, variously affecting the skin, lungs, or body as a whole.
Bleb	A small blister usually filled with blood or fluid.
Blepharitis	Inflammation of the eyelids, usually due to bacterial infection; sometimes associated with allergies or seborrhoea of the face and scalp.
Blind spot	A small spot on the retina, where the optic nerve enters, which is insensitive to light.
Blood-brain barrier	Some natural body substances, drugs, and chemicals circulating in the blood are unable to reach active brain cells. The apparent blood-brain barrier permits some substances to enter

and prevents others. It is thought by some authorities to consist of a layer of cells around small capillaries in the brain. The barrier is presumably a natural protective mechanism.

A general term for the presence of germs or their toxins in circulating blood. See BACTERAEMIA, SEPTICAEMIA, TOXAEMIA.

Blood poisoning

Laboratory tests of blood can yield a vast amount of information. The extent of testing depends on what is being looked for. There are many special tests for special purposes. A routine test does not include unusual procedures, but does include standard studies, for which the following are normal physiological values: pH (acid-alkaline ratios; pH 7 is neutral, above 7 is alkaline) 7·35 7·45   Red blood cells (erythrocytes)   4,500,000–5,000,000 per cu.mm.   White blood cells (leucocytes)   5,000 10,000 per cu.mm.   Polymorphonuclear neutrophils 60 70%   Lymphocytes 25 33%   Monocytes 2 6%   Eosinophils 1 3%   Basophils 0·25 0·5%   Platelets 200,000 400,000 per cu.mm.   Haemoglobin 14 16 gm per 100 ml.   Bleeding time 1 3 minutes   Coagulation time 6 12 minutes   Serum cholesterol 150 to 250 mg per 100 ml. .   Glucose 80 120 mg per 100 ml.   Albumin 3·5 5·5 gm per 100 ml.   Nonprotein nitrogen 25 38 mg per 100 ml.

Blood tests

An infant with a congenital heart defect which allows venous and arterial blood to mix, resulting in insufficient oxygen in the blood, producing blue skin and mucous membranes.

Blue baby

See SOMATOTYPE.

Body build

See SARCOIDOSIS.

Boeck's sarcoid

An index of physiological maturity, based on the fairly definite schedule of development of bone from birth to maturity, independent of chronological age. Bone age is commonly estimated by taking X-rays of a child's hands and wrists and comparing the centres of ossification with standards appropriate to his age. There are normal variations; bone age may be

Bone age

advanced or retarded a year or so without necessarily being abnormal. Advanced bone age may be associated with overactivity of the adrenal or thyroid glands, retarded bone age with deficient thyroid activity or malnutrition. Tall children who reach sexual maturity at an early age usually have advanced bone age; those who have retarded bone age are probably late maturers.

Bone banks

Stored collections of pieces of human bone. When transplanted, the dead sterile bone somehow stimulates the growth of new bone around it, eventually is incorporated into that new bone, and is slowly replaced. In the meantime the graft is a barrier which prevents soft fibrous tissue from filling the hole or defect in the patient's own bone. Bone grafts are used most frequently to correct curvature of the spine in children, and after fractures, if the bone ends fail to unite properly.

Bone conduction

Bones of the head are natural channels for conduction of sounds to the ears. This can be demonstrated by stopping the ears and touching a vibrating tuning fork to the skull or teeth. Some types of hearing aids, in contact with bone behind the ear, make use of this phenomenon. Bone conduction explains why our own voices do not sound the same to us as they do to others.

Bone marrow examination

Microscopic study of bone marrow tissue obtained by needle, used in diagnosing certain diseases of the blood.

Booster dose

Injection of a vaccine or immunizing agent given some time after an original vaccination to enhance its effectiveness. Immunizations tend to wear off in the course of time; a booster rejuvenates them. Some primary immunizations are given in two or three spaced injections, several days or weeks apart, to produce maximal immunizing action.

Bornholm disease
(*Devil's grip,
epidemic pleurodynia*)

An infectious disease of sudden onset, produced by COXSACKIE VIRUS, marked by knifelike pains in the chest or abdomen.

Botulism

A dangerous form of food poisoning caused by toxins of

botulinus organisms in improperly preserved foods. This disease is now seldom seen from food poisoning, but has recently arisen spontaneously in infants.

A slender cylindrical instrument introduced into a body orifice to explore or dilate a passage or act as a guide for other instruments.	**Bougie**
Bending of the middle joint of a finger with extension of the other joints, resulting from the cutting or rupture of a tendon.	**Boutonnière deformity**
Outward bowing of the knee joints; common in young children just beginning to walk, usually requiring no treatment unless bowing persists after five or six years of age.	**Bowlegs** (*genu varum*)
The cup-shaped capsule of a *nephron*, the minute filtering unit of the kidney.	**Bowman's capsule**
Abnormal slowness of the heartbeat, with a pulse rate of less than 60 per minute.	**Bradycardia**
Minute electric currents of brain cells which, when amplified and transcribed, have the form of spiked or wavy lines. See ELECTROENCEPHALOGRAPH.	**Brain waves**
A common source of breast pain, especially if the breasts are unusually large, is a poorly fitted brassiere which supports most of the weight from above by shoulder straps. Correct breast support sustains most of the weight of the breasts from *below*, by the portion of the brassiere which encircles the chest under the breasts; the main function of shoulder straps is to hold the garment in position.	**Breast support**
Crying of infants and small children so furious that they hold their breath until they turn blue or even lose consciousness for a moment. A breath-holding spell can be frightening the first time a parent is confronted with it, but the episode is just a bout of temper, and nature has arranged that we cannot hold our breath long enough to do serious harm.	**Breath-holding**

B

Breech delivery	Presentation of an infant's buttocks instead of the head at the outlet of the birth canal.
Bright's disease	An old term for several diseases which fall under the general category of *glomerulonephritis*.
Bromhidrosis	Foul-smelling perspiration, caused by decomposition of sweat and debris by bacteria.
Bromism	Chronic poisoning from long continued use of bromides; these drugs are now seldom used.
Bronchial tree	The breathing passages which extend from the windpipe in finer and finer ramifications.
Bronchiectasis	Dilatation of bronchial tubes usually a result of pus-producing infections or obstruction by foreign bodies.
Bronchitis	Inflammation of the linings of bronchial tubes.
Bronchography	The taking of an X-ray film of the lungs after injection of a radiopaque substance.
Bronchoscope	A tubelike instrument, inserted into the windpipe for purposes of inspecting tissues, withdrawing secretions or tissue samples, administering medicines, or extracting foreign bodies.
Bronzed diabetes	See HAEMOCHROMATOSIS.
Brucellosis	(*Malta fever, undulant fever*) An infectious disease transmitted from animals to man, most commonly by contact with cattle or consumption of raw milk products. Called *undulant fever*, from the type of fever. Recovery from acute brucellosis is usually spontaneous but convalescence may be prolonged. Chronic brucellosis may be unrecognized and hard to diagnose; varied symptoms – obscure fever of long duration, weakness, fatigability, excessive sweating – may puzzlingly resemble those of infectious mononucleosis, tuberculosis, malaria, or rheumatic fever. Positive diagnosis is made by recovery of brucella organisms from body excretions.

B

The habit of grinding the teeth.	**Bruxism**
A test for liver function.	**BSP**
An inflamed, swollen lymph node, usually in the groin or armpit, caused by absorption of infective materials.	**Bubo**
Of or relating to the cheek or mouth.	**Buccal**
Inflammation of the inner walls of blood vessels with clot formation and interruption of blood supply. The legs, feet, and toes are especially affected. Shutting off the blood supply can lead to GANGRENE and amputation. The cause of the disease is unknown but it chiefly affects young men and is almost never seen in nonsmokers. Absolute prohibition of smoking for the rest of the patient's life is an essential part of treatment; resumption of smoking can provoke renewed attacks and gangrene.	**Buerger's disease**
Insatiable appetite, requiring enormous meals for satisfaction.	**Bulimia**
A large blister.	**Bulla**
Enlargement and thickening of the big joint of the big toe, bending the big toe towards the little toe. The deformity becomes progressively worse if untreated. Surgical correction is not so simple as it seems, but is indicated for young persons. In older persons, a special shoe made to fit the deformity comfortably may be the most practical solution.	**Bunion** (*hallux valgus*)
Enlargement of the eye.	**Buphthalmos**
A form of malignant tumour, especially affecting the jaw and facial bones, most frequent in children of central Africa, but also occurring elsewhere. The tumour responds well to therapy. The disease is thought to be caused by a virus (Epstein-Barr).	**Burkitt's lymphoma**
A sac between opposing surfaces that slide past each other. It	**Bursa**

is filled with lubricating fluid, which permits free motion. Inflammation of a bursa causes painful *bursitis*, as of the shoulder, elbow, knee, or ankle.

Butterfly suture

A strip of plastic or adhesive tape with a relatively thin bridge between wider ends, used to draw together the opposing edges of a minor laceration on a smooth skin surface.

Byssinosis

An occupational disease of textile workers caused by inhalation of dusts produced during certain processing stages in cotton, flax, and hemp mills. Initial symptoms are chest tightness, cough, wheezing, and shortness of breath, which occur predominantly on the first working days after absence from work, as over a weekend. The cause is thought to be a chemical substance in textile dusts which constricts the bronchi and causes asthma-like symptoms.

C

Profound weakness, emaciation, general ill health, resulting from serious disease such as cancer.	**Cachexia**
The blind pouch in which the large bowel begins; the appendix projects from it.	**Caecum**
Delivery of a baby through an incision in the abdomen and uterus. Legend has it that Julius Caesar was born in this way.	**Caesarean section**
Multiple pigmented patches in the skin, the colour of coffee with milk, associated with NEUROFIBROMATOSIS.	**Cafe au lait spots**
A chemical substance contained in tea, coffee, and cola beverages. Caffeine is a powerful stimulant of the central nervous system and tends to increase both mental and physical performance. A great variety of drug preparations contain caffeine, often in combination with other drugs.	**Caffeine**
Divers' paralysis; cramping pain in the abdomen, legs, and other parts, called 'the bends' by divers. Symptoms are caused by nitrogen bubbles in the blood. The nitrogen gets into the blood from air inhaled under pressure, as under water or in caissons or wherever surrounding pressure greatly exceeds that of the atmosphere. Attacks can be prevented by gradual ascent from a deep dive, or treated by putting the patient into a decompression chamber where high pressure is gradually reduced while nitrogen slowly dissipates from body fluids. The bends can affect scuba divers who stay long under water at depths of 100 feet or so and ascend too rapidly.	**Caisson disease**
The heel bone.	**Calcaneus**
The process by which tissues become hardened by deposits of calcium salts.	**Calcification**
A mineral element that is an essential constituent of bone and is essential for blood clotting, muscle tone, and nerve function.	**Calcium**

Calculus

A stone formed in a duct, cyst, or hollow organ of the body, especially in the gallbladder and kidney. Most calculi are composed of mineral salts, often with a mixture of organic matter. The composition of a stone may sometimes give the doctor information of value in preventing future stone formation. Stones range in size from specks of sand to stones which fill the entire interior of the organ. The material that stones are made of is somehow extracted and condensed from fluids of the body. Infection and stagnation of fluids play a part in stone formation, but exactly why some people form stones and others do not, is not known. Drinking hard water is not a causative factor. Stones may cause few symptoms if they stay where they are, but severe pain ensues if a stone tries to squeeze through a passage too small for it. *Dental calculus* is tartar that accumulates on teeth.

Callus

A patch of hard, thickened skin, usually on the hands or feet; a protective reaction to pressure or friction. A callus is like a corn except that it is more diffuse and has no core, and it tends to disappear spontaneously when the cause is removed. Persons who stand a great deal often develop thick calluses of the heel or ball of the foot. The hard skin may be removed by rubbing with pumice stone, emery board, or a coarse Turkish towel after soaking the foot in hot water. Persistent calluses which cause a great deal of discomfort should have the attention of a chiropodist. Callus is also a word for the bony material which exudes from and surrounds broken bone ends and plays a part in the healing of a fracture.

Calorie

A unit of heat. The unit used in measuring body metabolism and the fattening propensities of foods is the large Calorie, the amount of heat necessary to raise the temperature of one kilogram of water one degree Centigrade. Nowadays the unit joule is preferred.

Calyx

One of the several small cuplike chambers which receive urine from the kidney tubules and channel it into the funnel-shaped cavity of the kidney which merges with the ureter.

Candidiasis

Infection caused by *Candida albicans*, which has a predilection for mucous membranes. Common sites of infection are the skin, nails, mouth, vagina, gastrointestinal tract. See vaginal yeast infections, in pregnancy, thrush.

A hollow tube for insertion into a body passage or cavity; within the cannula there is usually a *trocar*, a sliding rod with a pointed tip, designed to puncture a cavity and release fluid, after which the trocar is withdrawn and fluid drains through the cannula.
| **Cannula**

The angle formed where the eyelids meet at the outer or inner side.
| **Canthus**

The smallest size of blood vessel.
| **Capillary**

The primary fuel of muscular activity, the major source of energy we need for moving, working, acting, living. Carbohydrates occur as sugars and starches, in many complex forms; the starches are converted to sugar by the digestive process. Cereals, vegetables, and fruits are inexpensive carbohydrate foods which are major sources of food for much of the world's population. Carbohydrate is necessary to burn fats efficently, and it spares protein, which can be burned for energy if necessary but is more valuable for other purposes. Cellulose, the indigestible matter in many carbohydrate foods, supplies useful bulk in the intestines. Most of the carbohydrate in the body is stored in the liver and muscles in the form of glycogen (animal starch), but not much more than a day's needs are held in storage. As the supplies become depleted, hunger pangs remind us that it is time to replenish our energy reserves.
| **Carbohydrate**

Extremely cold snowlike particles about –73˚C (–100˚F) formed by rapid evaporation of liquid carbon dioxide. Application of the snow freezes the skin instantly. It is used in treatment of various skin lesions, such as birthmarks.
| **Carbon dioxide snow**

A colourless, odourless gas which can cause fatal poisoning. Immediate first aid is imperative. Carbon monoxide kills by depriving tissues of oxygen; it combines 200 times more readily than oxygen with HAEMOGLOBIN of the red blood cells. The gas
| **Carbon monoxide**

is produced by any incompletely burned fuel. A common belief that a fire in a closed space is dangerous because it burns up all the oxygen is erroneous; it is dangerous because it emits carbon monoxide. It is dangerous to let a car run in a closed garage even for seconds. Gas can also seep into a car from a leaky silencer or exhaust pipe. Relatively small amounts of the gas in a car driven with windows closed can dull a driver's senses or cause him to fall asleep at the wheel. It is wise to drive with one window at least partly open and to have the exhaust system checked for leaks during routine inspections.

Carbuncle	A deep-seated infection of the skin, like several boils joined together; pus is discharged from a number of points on the tight, reddened skin surface.
Carcinogen	Any agent which tends to produce cancer.
Carcinoma	Cancer comprised of epithelial cells, the type that cover the skin and mucous membranes and form the linings of organs. Carcinomas may arise in almost any structure of the body; many forms are curable if proper treatment is begun early.
Cardiac	Of or relating to the heart.
Cardiac asthma	(an undesirable term) Paroxysms of difficult breathing, often occurring at night, characteristic of congestive heart failure. It is a quite different condition from bronchial asthma.
Cardiac catheter	A slender tube which is threaded into a vessel of the arm and on into the heart to obtain several kinds of important diagnostic information.
Cardiac pacemaker	A device which electrically stimulates the heart, triggering the beat and producing contractions at or near the normal rate when the organ itself cannot do so reliably.
Cardiac sphincter	The valve of ringlike muscle at the junction of oesophagus and stomach.
Cardiospasm	See ACHALASIA.

Of or relating to the heart and blood vessels.	**Cardiovascular**
Decay of bone; the dentist's word for tooth decay (dental caries).	**Caries**
A yellow pigment occurring in carrots, leaves, yellow vegetables, egg yolk, and other foodstuffs. The body converts it into vitamin A. Excessive intake over a long period of time of carrots or other carotene-rich foods may raise the blood's content of carotene to such an exaggerated level that the skin takes on a yellowish hue, sometimes mistaken for jaundice. This condition, known as *carotenaemia*, is harmless.	**Carotene**
The principal artery that runs up each side of the neck. At approximately the middle of the neck it divides in a Y shape; one branch continues as the external carotid artery which goes to the face and scalp, and the other as the internal carotid artery which goes directly to the brain. Some strokes are caused by obstruction of the artery at the Y; the structure is close to the surface, readily accessible to a surgeon, and an operation may result in great improvement of the patient's symptoms. Overstimulation or compression of nerves at the point where the artery divides can cause dizziness and loss of consciousness.	**Carotid**
Of or relating to the wrist. The *carpal tunnel* through which a large nerve passes from the wrist to the hand may become constricted and cause tingling and numbness of the fingers.	**Carpal**
See MOTION SICKNESS	**Car sickness**
Gristle; white, elastic, connective tissue. It is the substance of soft parts of infants which later become bone. It forms part of the skeleton. Pads of cartilage cushion the opposing surfaces of joints; thinning or wearing away of cartilage is associated with some forms of arthritis. The stiff but flexible substance of the external ear is cartilage. Cartilage does not have a blood supply and if injured cannot heal. Tearing or other injury of cartilage is quite common among athletes. This often requires surgical removal of the cartilage, for example from the knee.	**Cartilage**

C

Caruncle	A small, nonmalignant, fleshy growth; a type which causes pain and bleeding (urethral caruncle) occurs at the urinary outlet of women, most frequently at the menopause.
Castration	Removal of the testicles or ovaries. Functional powers of both can be destroyed by radiation. Sometimes necessary in treatment of disease; this is called nonsurgical castration.
Casts *renal*	Shed material in sediments of urine, sometimes indicative of latent forms of kidney disease. There are four forms of casts, *hyaline* (glassy), *red cell*, *granular*, and *epithelial*, from which inferences concerning the nature of kidney lesions may be drawn.
Catabolism	The breaking-down aspect of METABOLISM; the breaking-down of complex substances by cells is often accompanied by release of energy. The opposite of ANABOLISM.
Cataract	An opacity of the lens of the eye. A cataract is not a foreign substance, but a biochemical change in structure. Babies may be born with cataracts and some of these cases are hereditary. Increasing age, physical injury, chemical injury from certain drugs and industrial chemicals, diabetes and other endocrine diseases, are associated with cataract formation, but the great majority of cataracts seem to be a part of the ageing process. The only way to restore useful vision is to remove the lens surgically; this permits light to enter the eye once again. Of course the light-bending powers and power of ACCOMMODATION of the absent lens are lost. The patient has to wear spectacles to replace the missing lens. He can see quite well again— a wonderful reprieve from partial or total blindness but it takes some adjustment and re-education. Many improvements have been and are being made in cataract glasses but they do not restore normal ease of seeing completely. Contact lenses have been improved and come closer to restoring normal visual function but are not suitable for everyone. Replacement of the opaque lens with a plastic substitute is becoming increasingly successful.
Catarrh	A flowing down; an old-fashioned term for inflammation of

C

mucous membranes, especially of the nose and throat, with free-flowing discharge, as in a cold.

A phase of schizophrenia in which the patient stands or sits in some fixed position for hours on end and resists all attempts to get him to speak or move.	**Catatonia**
A peculiar condition of infants who give a cry like that of a cat, because of defective development of the larynx. It is an inherited abnormality, resulting from lack of a short arm on one of the infant's CHROMOSOMES.	**Cat cry syndrome**
A purgative medicine; a substance that increases evacuation of the bowels. Regular use of cathartics is unwise; they can be habit-forming, and do not correct an underlying condition. Cathartics or laxatives should not be used if abdominal pain is present, and powerful cathartics such as castor oil or epsom salts should be used only as the doctor directs.	**Cathartic**
A hollow tube for insertion through a canal into a cavity to discharge fluids, especially of the urinary bladder. The heart may also be catheterized for diagnostic purposes.	**Catheter**
An infection characterized by painless swelling of lymph nodes, acquired from a scratch by a cat.	**Cat scratch disease**
The head of a baby born with a caul is covered with a fetal membrane, the AMNION, which has become detached.	**Caul**
Burning pain caused by injury to sensory nerves, especially of the palms and soles; often associated with poor circulation to the part and discoloration, clamminess, and coldness of the skin. Blocking the affected nerves with procaine may give relief.	**Causalgia**
Application of heat or a chemical to destroy tissue. In ancient times, a red hot iron was applied to wounds to stop bleeding and infection. Today the most common form is *electrocautery*, in which a wire loop heated by electric current is used to seal bleeding vessels or destroy tissue.	**Cautery**

C

Cellulitis

Diffuse septic inflammation of soft, loose connective tissue beneath the skin.

Cementum

The bonelike substance which covers the roots of teeth.

Centigrade (C)

A thermometer scale, in which water freezes at 0 degrees C and boils at 100 degrees C. To convert to Fahrenheit degrees, multiply degrees Centigrade by nine fifths and add 32. Average body temperature is 37° Centigrade (98.6° Fahrenheit).

Central nervous system (*CNS*)

The brain and nerves of the spinal cord. The system is central because it is the functional headquarters of the whole nervous system, and all the nerves of the body enter or leave the brain or spinal cord.

Cephalic

Of or relating to the head. Turning the fetus so that the head presents at the cervix is called *cephalic version*.

Cerebellum

A specialized part of the brain, underneath the CEREBRUM at the back of the head. It is concerned with equilibrium and coordination of movements.

Cerebral palsy

A form of paralysis manifested by jerky, writhing, spastic movements, resulting from damage to brain centre controls of muscles. Cerebral palsy is not a single disease but a group of syndromes with a common factor, some form of injury to motor control centres in the brain. It is not always possible to determine the cause of brain damage. It may result from birth injury, from infections of the mother or fetus, from errors of development, and other causes.

Cerebrospinal fluid

Clear colourless fluid that surrounds the spinal cord and is continuous with the same fluid in the ventricles of the brain. Examination of the fluid assists in the diagnosis of various diseases (such as meningitis, polio, brain tumour) which cause changes in the fluid. The fluid may contain blood, pus, and other abnormal constituents; it may be given chemical, microscopic, and bacteriological tests and may be cultured to determine the presence and identity of germs.

C

A stroke, resulting from interruption of blood supply to the brain. The cause may be obstruction by a clot of a vessel supplying the brain, or rupture of a vessel with bleeding into brain tissue.	**Cerebrovascular accident**
The main part of the brain; the great mass of nerve tissue that occupies the entire upper part of the skull. *Cerebral* refers to phenomena that occur in the cerebrum; for example, cerebral haemorrhage.	**Cerebrum**
Ear wax.	**Cerumen**
A rough spot in the membrane lining the opening of the cervix.	**Cervical erosion**
An extra rib in the cervical or neck region, in addition to the usual twelve on each side. It can sometimes be felt as a bony projection at the root of the neck. The rib may cause no trouble, but if pressure or other disturbing symptoms develop, it may require operation.	**Cervical rib**
Inflammation of the neck of the uterus.	**Cervicitis**
A neck; the word applies to any necklike or constricted part of the body; especially, the tapering neck of the uterus. Also, the neck of the urinary bladder. The seven cervical vertebrae constitute the topmost part of the spine; cervical lymph nodes occur in the neck region.	**Cervix**
A blue discoloration around the entrance to the vagina and on the neck of the uterus; an early indication of pregnancy.	**Chadwick's sign**
See INTERTRIGO.	**Chafing**
A painless small tumour or cyst of the eyelid due to an obstructed drainage duct; dammed-up secretions cause the swelling. Hot compresses can be applied, together with an antibacterial medicine if the doctor so directs. If the tumour does not disappear spontaneously incision may be necessary.	**Chalazion**

Chancre	The primary lesion of syphilis; a hard sore or ulcer at the site where syphilis germs gained entrance to the body.
Chancroid (*soft chancre*)	A nonsyphilitic venereal disease caused by a specific bacillus, *Haemophilus ducreyi*. Initially a soft sore appears, usually on the genitals. In a few days it breaks down into a painful pus-discharging ulcer.
Chemotherapy	Treatment with chemicals which favourably alter the course of a disease.
Cheyne-Stokes respiration	An abnormal form of breathing in some patients with heart, kidney, or vascular disease. Intensity of breathing gradually decreases until no breath at all is taken for a few seconds or longer. This is followed by increase in breathing and shortage of breath. The pattern occurs in repeated cycles. One of the causes is thought to be a decrease in blood supply to the brain.
Chilblain (*erythema pernio*)	An acute or chronic form of cold injury, less severe than frostbite, characterized by inflammation of the skin, itching and swelling, frequently followed by blisters. The immediate cause is exposure to cold, to which some persons have an exaggerated sensitivity; it is advisable for them to stay indoors or wear heavy garments and fleece-lined gloves and overshoes during cold weather. Such persons should begin to wear protective clothing early in the winter when the environmental temperature drops below 15°C(60°F).
Chloasma	Discoloration of the skin with yellow-brown spots and patches. The condition is often associated with some endocrine disturbance. Chloasma frequently occurs in pregnancy as a result of increased secretion of a pituitary hormone, MSH, which stimulates pigment-producing cells. Hormone production returns to a normal level soon after delivery and the pigmented areas fade, though not always completely.
Chocolate cysts	Cysts of the ovary filled with chocolate-coloured material, characteristic of *endometriosis*.

Inflammation of the bile ducts.	**Cholangitis**
Inflammation of the gallbladder. It may occur in acute or chronic forms.	**Cholecystitis**
Stones in the gallbladder or its ducts.	**Cholelithiasis**

A serious epidemic infectious disease caused by comma-shaped germs transmitted in bowel discharges of carriers to food and water. It is characterized by profuse watery diarrhoea, cramps, vomiting, prostration, and suppression of urine. The principal by which cholera weakens and kills is through extreme losses of body fluids and ELECTROLYTES. Trravellers going to regions where cholera outbreaks occur (India, Pakistan, South East Asia) should be vaccinated with a cholera vaccine which gives some immunity for about six months.

Cholera

A mass that forms in the middle of the middle ear. The first sign may be a scanty discharge from the ear when the mass liquefies and perforates the drum. This also causes erosion of bone, which may extend dangerously into neighbouring structures. In most cases, surgical removal of the cholesteatoma is the best treatment.

Cholesteatoma

A waxy substance resembling fat in its properties, closely related to the sex hormones and vitamin D. It is present in all animal tissues. It regulates the passage of substances through cell walls, keeps us from becoming waterlogged when we bathe, and prevents us from losing too much water from evaporation. It is so important to the body that it is manufactured by the liver and other tissues whether we get cholesterol in our diets or not. Despite these virtues, cholesterol has become something of a scare word, blamed for degenerating the walls of arteries and setting the stage for heart attacks. However, most specialists are reluctant to indict cholesterol as the predominant factor in heart and blood vessel diseases. One reason for cholesterol's bad publicity is that it is easier for doctors to measure than other fatty components of blood serum. Clinically, such measurement is useful as an index of

Cholesterol

the overall pattern of fatty substances in the blood. The normal range of serum cholesterol is about 125 to 265 mg per 100 ml. It tends to rise in later years, and changes can be caused by variations in thyroid activity, diabetes, kidney insufficiency, and stress. Moderation of fat intake, reduction of weight if obese, and substitution of polyunsaturated fats for some of the hard fats in the diet are prudent measures in the present state of knowledge.

Chondroma	A tumour with the structure of CARTILAGE, usually benign, but with a tendency to recur after removal.
Chorea	A disease of the nervous system manifested by involuntary, irregular, rapid, jerky movements of muscles of the face, legs, and arms. Its common form (also called *St. Vitus' dance* and *Sydenham's chorea*) is a disease of childhood, often a manifestation of rheumatic fever. The jerky movements and facial grimaces subside in a few weeks. Signs of rheumatic disease may never appear, but about half the patients with chorea develop or have rheumatic fever. HUNTINGTON'S CHOREA is an entirely different hereditary disease.
Chorion	The outermost of the fetal membranes. The fetal part of the placenta develops from it.
Choroid	The middle coat of the eye, continuous with the iris in front; a thin, pigmented layer composed largely of interlaced blood vessels, vital to the eye's nutrition.
Christmas disease	A hereditary bleeding disease, having the same symptoms as classic haemophilia but resulting from deficiency of a different blood-clotting factor. Named after the family in whom it was discovered.
Chromosomes	Threadlike bodies in the nucleus of a cell; they contain the GENES and DNA.
Chronic	Long continued ill health as opposed to *acute* illness.
Cilia	Minute hairlike processes of specialized cells which beat rhythmically and keep debris-laden fluids flowing in one direction; for example, out of the lungs. The word also means eyelashes.

C

The part of the eye which suspends the lens and secretes aqueous humour.	**Ciliary body**
Cycles and rhythms of body processes that recur approximately every 24 hours. See BIOLOGICAL CLOCKS.	**Circadian rhythms**
Removal of the foreskin or prepuce of the penis.	**Circumcision**
Chronic, progressive inflammation of the liver, with increase of nonfunctioning fibrous tissue, distortion of liver cells, enlargement or shrivelling of the organ, and various eventual complications such as oedema, digestive complaints, weight loss, jaundice, bleeding veins of the oesophagus.	**Cirrhosis of the liver**
Puncture at a point beneath the skull in the back of the neck to withdraw CEREBROSPINAL FLUID, when the more usual method of lumbar puncture is not possible.	**Cisternal puncture**
Lameness, limping. *Intermittent claudication*, characterized by cramplike pain in the legs which comes on when walking, is usually a symptom of obliterative arterial disease.	**Claudication**
The collarbone.	**Clavicle**
Congenital malformation of structures of the lip, palate, or both, which fail to fuse properly during fetal development. The bilateral parts of the lips and palate normally fuse at about the eighth week of pregnancy.	**Cleft lip, -palate**
The change of life. See MENOPAUSE and MALE CLIMACTERIC.	**Climacteric**
Of or relating to the bedside; by extension, observation and treatment of patients, results and experience thus gained, as opposed to theoretical, laboratory, or experimental medicine.	**Clinical**
The small erectile sex organ of the female, situated above the vagina; homologue of the penis.	**Clitoris**
A drug that lowers fat levels in the blood, prescribed in the	**Clofibrate**

hope that such lowering may reduce the incidence of heart attacks.

Clonic

Spasmodic muscular contractions and relaxations which succeed each other alternately and jerkily. It may be combined with *tonic* contractions which are continuous.

Clonorchis

A chronic Asiatic disease caused by liver flukes transmitted by raw, smoked, or pickled fish.

Clubbed fingers

Short, broad, bulbous finger ends with overhanging nails. The condition results from local deficiency of oxygenated blood and is usually associated with abnormalities of the heart and respiratory system such as congenital heart malformation, emphysema, bronchiectasis, chronic disease of the heart and chest.

Clubfoot (*talipes*)

A foot twisted out of shape so that the sole does not rest flat on the floor when standing; there are several types. Heredity has little if anything to do with the condition. The principal causative factor is thought to be a fixed position of the fetus in the uterus maintained for a long period of fetal life; scantiness of amniotic fluid possibly inhibits free movement of the fetus. Pressures of long-maintained fixed posture tend to modify the development of body parts in a mechanical way.

Coagulation time

The time it takes a sample of blood to form a clot, determined by laboratory procedures. This information is useful in treating patients with a tendency to haemorrhage, and as a guide to treatment of patients receiving anticoagulants.

Coarctation of the aorta

Congenital constriction of the great vessel which carries arterial blood from the heart.

Cobalt bomb

In medicine, not really a bomb but a device employing radioisotopes of cobalt for powerful irradiation of patients, usually suffering from cancer.

Coccus

A small round bacterium. Some types, such as those which cause gonorrhoea and pneumonia, occur in pairs; other types form chains and others cluster in irregular masses like bunches of grapes.

The fused vertebrae at the tip of the spine; the tailbone.	**Coccyx**
A bony pea-sized structure of the inner ear, shaped like a snail shell, lined with fine hairs and nerve endings which are the essential organs of the sense of hearing.	**Cochlea**
A disorder, believed to have a hereditary basis, in which the small intestine is unable to absorb fat from foods. See MALAB-SORPTION SYNDROME.	**Coeliac disease**
A partner needed by some enzymes to accomplish a biochemical change. Many vitamins are coenzymes.	**Coenzyme**
Dark brown or blackish granular vomited material, somewhat resembling coffee grounds; the colour comes from changed blood and indicates slow bleeding in the upper digestive tract.	**Coffee-ground vomit**
Sexual intercourse.	**Coitus**
A drug prepared from roots of the meadow saffron which is specific in relieving acute attacks of GOUT.	**Colchicine**

Fibres in the connective tissue which supports the body; it constitutes 40 per cent in the body's protein. In ways not fully understood, it is associated with rheumatic and other diseases, collectively called collagen or connective tissue diseases. Collagen fibres vary greatly in structure and function. Some, as in the cornea of the eye, are transparent. Collagen is the cushioning material of cartilage in the joints, the matrix on which minerals are laid down to form bones, the inelastic material of tendons which transfer muscle movements over joints, the elastic part of skin, a part of webs and struts which hold the body together, a substance which when boiled yields glue or gelatine. Once laid down in the body, collagen is not renewed or replaced. Old collagen is less elastic than young collagen. It is related to stiffness of joints and laxity of skin with

Collagen

increasing age, and may be a good index of a person's biological rather than chronological age.

Collapsed lung	Pneumothorax or atelectasis.

Colles' fracture

A common fracture of one of the forearm bone (*radius*) near the wrist joint on the thumb side. It is usually a consequence of falling with an arm thrust out and hand bent backward to break the fall.

Colloid goitre

Soft, smooth, symmetrical enlargement of the thyroid, usually as a result of iodine deficiency; simple goitre.

Colon

The large bowel.

Colostomy

A surgically created opening of the colon (artificial anus) in the wall of the abdomen. A colostomy may be temporary, to divert intestinal contents while a portion of the colon is healing, or it may be permanent, as is usually the case if a large section of the bowel must be removed because of disease. A *colostomy bag* is a container which covers the artificial opening and receives excretions.

Colostrum

The first milk secreted by the mother's breasts shortly after the birth of a child. Colostrum is not true milk but a clear or slightly cloudy fluid containing fats and sugars which have a slight laxative effect on the newborn baby. Colostrum also contains IMMUNOGLOBULINS which pass on to the baby some of the immunities acquired by the mother; this immunity is not long lasting.

Colour blindness

Inability to distinguish colours. There are many types and degrees of colour blindness, some so slight that an affected person may never be aware of it. Colour blindness does not affect keeness of vision and is no great handicap except in occupations where safety or fine colour discrimination is important. A colour blind man may choose a shirt, tie, jacket, socks, and trousers of violently clashing hues. Total colour blindness in which everything is seen as shades of grey is rare. The most common type is red-green colour blindness, which may range from ability to see only the brightest hues of red and green to inability to see the two colours as other than shades of grey. Injury to the retina or ocular disease may produce colour blindness, but this is very rare. Colour blindness is almost always inherited; a few women are partially colour blind but the condition predominantly affects the male sex. Common red-green colour blindness is a sex-linked trait, transmitted to her sons but not her daughters by a mother who herself is not colour blind. The inherited defect is in the structure of the CONES, the colour-sensitive nerve cells of the retina. Nothing can be done to change the defect, although some improvement in discrimination of shades may be attained by training.

Any surgical cutting of the vagina.	**Colpotomy**
Unconsciousness so deep that it is impossible or extremely difficult to rouse the patient. Many different conditions cause coma; advanced liver and kidney disease, diabetes, poisoning, head blows, tumours, strokes, to mention a few.	**Coma**
Blackhead	**Comedo**
One in which the bone is broken into pieces.	**Comminuted fracture**
One in which the broken bone breaks through the skin or into an open wound.	**Compound fracture**
Violent jarring, shocking, shaking, or the resulting condition. *Concussion of the brain* may result from a fall or violent blow on the head. The injured person may not be knocked out, but may be dizzy, sleepy, nauseated, or he may lose consciousness and have a feeble pulse, cold skin, and pallor. Medical help should be sought immediately, even though the person seems to have recovered or to be only slightly dazed. A doctor treating concussion may wish to keep the patient under observation, or to make tests, to be sure that the skull has not been fractured, or the brain damaged.	**Concussion**
Failure of airborne sound waves to be conducted efficiently	**Conduction deafness**

through and over the external and middle ear structures, so that adequate messages do not reach the nerves of the inner ear.

Condyloma

A warty growth on the skin around the anus and external sex organs.

Cones

Specialized cells of the central part of the retina which distinguish colours and are responsible for finely detailed vision.

Congenital malformations

Abnormalities that are present at birth. See BIRTH DEFECTS.

Conization

Reaming out of a cone-shaped piece of tissue by high-frequency current; usually a gynaecological procedure performed on a diseased cervix.

Conjunctiva

The thin mucous membrane which covers the insides of the eyelids and is reflected over the front of the eye. *Conjunctivitis* is an inflammation of this tissue resulting from infection, allergies, irritation, or inflammation from within the eye itself.

Consanguinity

Blood relationship

Contact dermatitis

Skin eruption, redness, or inflammation, resulting from contact with any of hundreds of substances.

Contact lenses

Plastic or glass lenses worn over the cornea of the eye. Meticulous fitting to the eye contours is essential. The lenses must have proper hygienic care. Serious complications are rare, minor ones not uncommon. The most painful complication appears to result from wearing the lenses too long. They should not be worn while sleeping, or when the eye is infected, or when there are cold sores on the face (the cold sore virus can infect the eyes dangerously). Flush-fitting contact lenses which cover the white of the eye permit a thin layer of tears to circulate beneath them and have special medical uses as healing aids. Such lenses improve the healing of chemical burns of the cornea, ulcerations, corneal transplants, and other conditions. Plastic lenses which absorb moisture have become available; see SOFT CONTACT LENSES.

Prevention of conception or impregnation.	**Contraception**
A medical term meaning that something is undesirable, or should not be done; for example alcohol is contraindicated in extreme cold.	**Contraindication**
A substance which has greater density to X-rays than tissues which are objects of study. Contrast media are given by injection or other means to obtain clearly outlined X-ray images of structures being examined.	**Contrast medium**
A bruise.	**Contusion**
An antibody test on blood, used in determining the compatibility of bloods for transfusion and in diagnosis of certain anaemias.	**Coombs' test**
The curved transparent tissue covering the iris and pupil on the outside of the eye; the window of the eye.	**Cornea**
The cornea may become scarred or clouded, obstructing vision. If the rest of the eye is in good condition, sight may be restored by transplanting a disc taken from the cornea of a recently deceased person. It is like replacing an opaque pane of glass with a transparent one. The procedure requires a supply of donor eyes, and eye banks have been established in many cities to receive and preserve donated eyes, which must be removed promptly after death of the donor. It is useless to donate one's eyes in a will, because of legal delays. Anyone wishing to donate his eyes after death should do so through his doctor or an eye bank.	**Corneal transplant**
Rough skin thickenings about the size of peas which occur principally on or between the toes. Soft corns between the toes are softened by sweat. The common hard corn has a cone-shaped core which presses on nerves to cause dull discomfort or sharp pain. Corns are caused by continued pressure and friction, as from too tight or illfitting shoes and stockings. Pressure can be relieved by wearing softer shoes with ample toe-room and by foam rubber pads and inserts. The hard tissue	**Corns**

of a corn usually must be removed as required for comfort's sake. Soaking the feet in hot water and paring the surface of the corn with a razor blade often relieves friction and pressure, but there is a risk of cuts and infection. Superficial hard tissue may be removed with an emery board, nail file, or pumice stone. The core may be sufficiently loosened by soaking to be lifted out by sterilized tweezers. Corn plasters and medicines usually contain salicylic acid which softens the hard growth. Diabetics should be especially careful in care of the feet because of the risk of ulcers.

Coronary thrombosis	Commonly called a heart attack; a blood clot in a coronary artery of the heart.
Cor pulmonale	A form of heart disease secondary to chronic disease of the lungs.
Corpuscle	Any small round body; the word used to be a synonym for cell. Technically, a cell has a nucleus; the mature red blood cell does not, and is sometimes called a corpuscle.
Corpus luteum	The yellow body which develops from a follicle of the ovary after a ripened egg has been discharged. The yellow body produces progesterone, a hormone which prepares the lining of the uterus to receive a fertilized egg. If fertilization occurs, the corpus luteum enlarges and continues to produce pregnancy-sustaining hormone for several months. If conception does not occur, the corpus luteum shrinks and degenerates.
Cortex	The surface layer of an organ such as the brain, kidney, adrenal gland. The cortex of an organ has different functions from its inner part (medulla); for example, the adrenal cortex produces hormones entirely different from those of its inner part. The thin surface layer of the brain (*cortex cerebri*) consists of grey matter, largely composed of small-bodied nerve cells with rich interconnections, interspersed with larger neurons which send AXONS into underlying white matter.
Corticosteroids	Substances having the properties of hormones secreted by the cortex of the adrenal glands. Cortisone, hydrocortisone, pred-

nisone, and many other corticosteroids have important medical uses.

An old word for the common cold.	**Coryza**
Inflammation of the skin, usually allergic, produced by contact with cosmetic creams, dyes, lotions, perfumes and the like.	**Cosmetic dermatitis**
Two small glands of the male which secrete lubricating fluids into the urethra.	**Cowper's glands**
A disease of cattle, so closely related to smallpox, and so mild in man, that inoculation with vaccine containing cowpox virus has long been the standard method of immunizing against smallpox.	**Cowpox**
A family of viruses named after a community in New York from whom the viruses were first isolated and identified. A score or more of different Coxsackie viruses cause diseases such as HERPANGINA, BORNHOLM DISEASE, and forms of *meningitis*.	**Coxsackie viruses**
Infestation by pubic lice.	**Crabs**
Patchy areas of greasy crusts on an infant's scalp, arising from secretions of oil glands.	**Cradle cap**
A nerve attached directly to the brain, leaving it through a perforation in the skull. There are twelve pairs of cranial nerves, with names that suggest their function or location: transmission of the sense of smell (*olfactory*), sight (*optic*), hearing (*acoustic*); control of movement of the eyeball (*trochlear*), a muscle of the eyeball (*abducens*), the pupil (*oculomotor*), muscles of the upper throat and taste sensations from the back of the tongue (*glossopharyngeal*), sense of taste, salivary glands and muscles of the face (*facial*), muscles of the larynx and throat (*accessory*), the tongue (*hypoglossal*); sensory nerve of the face and front part of the scalp (*trigeminal*); sensory and motor nerve branching to the heart, stomach, and oesophagus (*vagus*).	**Cranial nerve**

C

Craniotomy	Surgical opening of the skull cavity.
Cranium	The skull.
Creeping eruption (*larvae migrans*)	A parasitic infection of the skin: thin, red, tortuous lines creep ahead at one end an inch or more a day while fading at the other end. The moving lines mark the progress of larvae burrowing under the skin. The burrowers, often immature forms of cat or dog hookworm, get into people who go barefoot on beaches, children in sandpits, gardeners, and repairmen who work under porches of houses. Freezing the larvae in the skin with an ethyl chloride spray usually stops their migrations.
Creeping ulcer	One which creeps slowly outward from its centre.
Cremaster	The muscle which retracts the testicle.
Cretin	A child born with an underactive thyroid gland.
Crohn's disease	See REGIONAL ILEITIS.
Crossed eyes	Eyes that do not work as a pair in holding the gaze straight on an object, because of imbalance of muscles that control movements of the eyeballs. An eye that turns in or out in young children may lose its vision completely unless the condition is corrected before it is too late.
Croup	Difficult laborious breathing and coughing of a child. *Spasmodic croup* is more frightening than serious; another type, *laryngotracheobronchitis*, is one of the most serious conditions of infancy and is a medical emergency.
Crowning	The stage in childbirth when the crown or top of the infant's head first becomes visible in the dilated outlet of the vagina.
Cryosurgery	Use of extreme cold to destroy or to freeze and later revive tissues. Pioneering cryosurgical work was done in the field of brain surgery, especially in surgical management of *Parkin-*

son's disease. Complete destruction of tissue by super-freezing has been used to relieve benign or malignant obstruction of the *prostate* gland. The freeze treatment for *gastric ulcer* does not permanently destroy stomach tissue, but tends to decrease acid production; longterm benefits are considered disappointing by many. A newer application of cryosurgery (more exactly, cryotherapy, since tissue is not destroyed) is in the treatment of *glaucoma*. The purpose is to decrease production of fluid in the eye. Cryotherapy is a reserve method if drugs or surgery fail to stop the advance of glaucoma.

A cavity, pit, or follicle; such as the natural depressions in the tonsils.	**Crypt**
Failure of the testicles to descend into the scrotum during fetal development; the undescended organs remain in the abdominal cavity or groin.	**Cryptorchidism**
Scraping out of a body cavity with a spoon-shaped instrument called a *curette*.	**Curettage**
An ulcer of the stomach or duodenum, associated with severe skin burns.	**Curling's ulcer**
Disorders resulting from excessive output of certain adrenal hormones.	**Cushing's syndrome**
The dead outer layer of skin; the crescent of skin at the base of nails.	**Cuticle**
A bluish tinge of the skin and mucous membranes resulting from insufficent oxygen in the blood. There are many different causes; for example, congenital heart defects, congestive heart failure, emphysema, mountain sickness, respiratory and blood disorders. The lips or the beds of the nails may sometimes take on a bluish discoloration without a deficiency of oxygen in the general circulation, simply from slow circulation due to cold.	**Cyanosis**
Pregnancy.	**Cyesis**

Cyst

A normal or abnormal sac with a definite wall, containing liquid or semisolid material. Frequent sites of cysts that may require surgery or other measures are the ovaries, kidneys, skin, the coccygeal area (pilonidal cyst), and breast.

Cysticercosis

Infestation of the body with tapeworm larvae, sometimes present in raw beef. Beef should be cooked at least to the rare stage (60°C, 140°F) to avoid danger.

Cystic fibrosis

An inherited disease of the *exocrine* glands which pour secretions into or out of the body rather than into the blood; for example, the pancreas and bilary, intestinal, and sweat glands. Thick viscid secretions obstruct or depress the functioning of many different organs and tissues and produce a variety of symptoms; respiratory distress is prominent. Cystic fibrosis was discovered in 1938, at which time it was thought to be a disease of the pancreas; it is known that nearly all the exocrine glands are affected to some degree. The earliest sign of cystic fibrosis in a newborn infant is MECONIUM ILEUS. Prompt recognition and treatment of cystic fibrosis, with aerosol aids for breathing, postural drainage, digestive enzymes, and antibiotics to combat infection, have carried affected infants through critical periods of childhood. The disease is being increasingly recognized in adults who have had it from infancy without realizing it. Doctors think it likely that many patients treated for bronchial asthma or various chronic lung conditions actually have a cystic fibrosis. The disease is transmitted as a recessive trait (the mother and father are carriers but do not have the disease themselves). An abnormal protein in the blood serum of cystic fibrosis patients and of blood-related persons is the possible basis for a test to detect carriers of the trait; if two carriers marry, the chance that each of their children will have cystic fibrosis is one in four.

Cystinuria

An inherited disease in which cystine, a sulphur-containing amino acid, is excreted in large quantities in the urine. The poorly soluble cystine tends to form recurrent kidney stones; alkalinizing the urine and drinking large amounts of water help to reduce the likelihood of cystine stone formation.

C

Sagging of the base of the bladder into the vaginal canal.	**Cystocele**
An instrument for examining the interior of the urinary bladder.	**Cystoscope**
Microscopic study of cells shed by body tissues to detect abnormalities, especially the presence of cancer cells. The PAPANICOLAOU SMEAR test for detection of cancer of the cervix is the most widely used cytological screening test, but the technique is applicable to smears obtained from the lungs, stomach, bladder, and a number of other organs.	**Cytological diagnosis**
Scientific study of the structure, elements, and function of cells.	**Cytology**
The substance of a cell outside its nucleus.	**Cytoplasm**
Drugs that are poisonous to body cells. Cancer cells are often more vulnerable to such drugs than normal tissues, and so these drugs have a valuabie part to play in the treatment of some kinds of cancer.	**Cytotoxic drugs**

D

Dilatation and curettage, a common minor operation on women; the canal of the uterus is dilated and the lining of the uterus scraped with a spoon-shaped instrument called a curette.	**D & C**
Fine, whitish, somewhat greasy scales formed upon the scalp; the condition is controllable but rarely curable.	**Dandruff**
Inability to hear and speak. The two disabilities are interrelated. A totally deaf child cannot learn to speak in the normal way because he cannot hear sounds to imitate. Various signs may arouse suspicion of deafness in an infant as young as six months. While the child is still young, he can be taught to speak by training techniques used in special schools for the deaf.	**Deaf-mutism**
Surgical cleaning of a wound; removal of foreign material and dead tissue.	**Débridement**
The withdrawal of calcium from the bones where it has been deposited. It may be caused by an inadequate supply of calcium in the diet so that calcium has to be taken from the bones, or by hormonal imbalances.	**Decalcification**
The unit of measurement of the loudness of sound, used in tests of hearing. A whisper is about twenty decibels loud.	**Decibel**
That part of the lining of the uterus which is modified during pregnancy and cast off after delivery.	**Decidua**
See PRESSURE SORES.	**Decubitus ulcer**
Passage of faeces; evacuation of the bowels.	**Defaecation**
Those caused by insufficiency of some constituent of the diet, such as vitamins, minerals, protein, fatty acids.	**Deficiency diseases**
The act of swallowing.	**Deglutition**
A splitting open, as of a sutured wound.	**Dehiscence**

Dehydration

Drying out of the body; loss of more water than is taken in. Dehydration may be induced for medical reasons, but often it is an aspect of disease or injury, characterized by dry mucous membranes, fever, scanty urine, soft or even wrinkled skin, possible shock. Treatment, which may present an emergency, requires recognition of underlying circumstances, calculation of water and ELECTROLYTE deficits, and usually replacement of water and salts (sometimes of plasma or blood) by infusion into a vein.

Déjà vu

Already seen; an illusion that a present experience has occurred at some previous time.

Delirium

A state of mental confusion, excitement, incoherent talk, restlessness, hallucinations. Delirium may be associated with high fever, poisoning, drug intoxication, infections, and metabolic disturbances. Treatment is directed to the underlying condition while the patient is kept in a quiet room, and closely watched to prevent injury. Tranquillizers may be prescribed. Reassurance by a close member of the family may help significantly to allay fears.

Delirium tremens (D.T.'s)

A serious, sometimes fatal form of delirium, most often occurring in persons with a long history of alcoholism, but occasionally associated with other poisoning of the brain cells, senile brain changes, and psychoses. The patient has vivid visual hallucinations, often of moving coloured animals, large or small; he may feel as well as see them crawling over his skin. Anxiety, fear, coarse trembling of the hands, mental confusion, and sleeplessness are other manifestations. Physical restraints may be necessary but skilful attendants can often avoid this. The delirium lasts for a couple of days to a week or more and usually terminates in deep sleep. The patient is often malnourished and run down physically. Appropriate tranquillizers and large doses of B vitamins are commonly a part of treatment. KORSAKOFF'S PSYCHOSIS may begin as delirium tremens.

Deltoid

Triangular in shape, like the Greek letter *delta*; specifically, the muscle which covers the shoulder joint and extends the arm out from the side.

D

A general term for mental deterioration, usually implying serious impairment of intellect, irrationality, confusion, stupor, insane behaviour. Dementia may result from poisons, physical changes in the brain, toxins produced by disease, or psychoses of which the basic cause is unknown. — **Dementia**

Fine, branched fibres, which accept and convey incoming impulses to the central body of a nerve cell. — **Dendrites**

Sudden high fever, called breakbone for the severe pain it causes in muscles, bones, and joints. It is not a dangerous disease. — **Dengue**

Replacement of lost teeth, as by reimplantation of a knocked-out tooth. — **Dental implants**

A thin, transparent film that builds up on the teeth. It is made up of material from saliva. The plaque contains bacteria which are thought to be a factor in tooth decay. — **Dental plaque**

The ivory-like material, harder and denser than bone, which underlies the enamel of the teeth. — **Dentine**

The set of natural teeth; also, a set of artificial teeth; 'false teeth'. — **Denture**

Sore mouth due to ill-fitting dentures or allergy to substances in the plates. — **Denture stomatitis**

Removal of hair. Permanent removal of unwanted hair is best accomplished by ELECTROLYSIS, which destroys the hair follicle. — **Depilation**

A single injection technique for desensitization to allergens, using oily emulsions. — **Depot desensitization**

Thickening of the sheaths covering the tendons of the thumb, resulting in pain at the base of the thumb, and radiating to the nail and into the forearm. Surgery corrects the condition, or it may cure itself if the wrist is immobilized. — **DeQuervain's disease** (*stenosing tenovaginitis*)

Dercum's disease
(*adiposis dolorosa*)

A rare disease of middle-aged and older women. Firm fat nodules, slightly sensitive or very painful, are distributed over various parts of the body except the face, lower arms, and lower legs; the overlying skin is red and shiny. There is pronounced muscular weakness and degree of psychological disturbance. The cause is not known. Nonspecific methods of treatment include measures to relieve pain, reduce weight, and combat the mental disturbances that may be associated.

Dermabrasion

A method of removing layers of skin with an abrasive instrument, usually a rapidly rotating wire brush, for cosmetic improvement of scars or blemishes.

Dermatitis

Inflammation of the skin. Its causes are manifold, its symptoms varied. Chemicals, plants, common household agents, cosmetics, drugs, X-rays, and many other things can produce dermatitis; allergies to various substances are often involved.

Dermatoglyphics

The study of the ridges, whorls, lines, and creases which form highly individual patterns of the skin of the hands and feet. Skin patterns determined by GENES begin to form in the fetus at about the fourth month of pregnancy. Several abnormal patterns, such as a single crease instead of the usual two which run across the top of the palm, are characteristic of infants with congenital disease. Some disorders such as MONGOLISM and KLINEFELTER'S SYNDROME result from abnormal CHROMO-SOMES. Others, such as malformations associated with the mother's infection by German measles, result from unfavourable environment of the fetus at the time when skin patterns as well as organ systems are developing. It is not yet possible to identify specific diseases by abnormal palmprints, but they usually indicate some congenital abnormality. Palmprint studies may give early warning of a congenital disorder, or confirm some suspected condition, such as mongolism, without the need for analyzing chromosomes.

Dermatome

An instrument for cutting thin layers of skin for grafts.

Dermatomyositis

An ill-defined disease of unknown cause, affecting connective tissue, manifested principally in the skin and voluntary muscles; characterized by pain and swelling in muscles, weakness, inflammation and swelling of skin of the face, upper trunk, and extremities.

Fungi which produce blistery, scaly, crusty lesions of the skin; most notoriously those responsible for *dermatophytosis* or athlete's foot.	**Dermatophytes**
The true skin, as opposed to the epidermis; the *corium*; a dense elastic layer of fibrous tissue underlying the topmost epithelial layers.	**Dermis**
Skin writing; a condition in which a tracing made on the skin by a fingernail or blunt instrument produces a pale streak bordered on each side by a reddened line. The marks disappear after a few minutes. The condition may be associated with NETTLE RASH but in itself is not injurious to health. Dermographia occurs in persons whose mechanisms for expanding and constricting blood vessels are sensitive to any irritation.	**Dermographia**
A congenital cyst (often of the ovary) which contains fragments of skin appendages such as strands of hair, sweat and oil glands, and sometimes cartilage, bone, and teeth, remnants of development.	**Dermoid cyst**
Reduction of a person's allergic reaction to a specific substance such as pollen or house dust. Sensitivity is reduced by spaced injections of small amounts of extracts of specific allergens; hay fever injections are a familiar example.	**Desensitization**
Shedding of the skin in scales or sheets, as after scarlet fever or severe sunburn.	**Desquamation**
Separation of the light-receiving layer of the back of the eye from its underlying layer. In the majority of cases, the detached filmy structure can be welded back into place by surgical procedures.	**Detached retina**
Diversion from a straight line of the bony wall that divides the	**Deviated septum**

nose into two equal parts, usually a result of injury but sometimes congenital. The deformity may not be obvious from the outside. Depending on its nature, a deviated septum may partially obstruct air passages, deflect air currents, and lead to mouth-breathing and profuse, annoying postnasal drip.

Dextrocardia	Congenital transposition of the axis of the heart towards the right of the chest.
Dextrose (*glucose*)	A sugar which is a source of energy, and necessary for combustion of fats. The liver converts dextrose into *Glycogen* (animal starch) and stores it. This reservoir is drawn upon for dextrose, reconverted from glycogen, as energy needs of the body require. Dextrose solutions are often infused into the veins of patients.
Dhobi itch	See TINEA CRURIS.
Diabetes	The word comes from a Greek term for syphon, or to flow through, referring to the excessive flow of urine and excessive thirst. Used alone, diabetes means *diabetes mellitus* or sugar diabetes. There are other forms of diabetes, such as *diabetes insipidus*, a hormone imbalance causing enormous thirst and compensating urinary outflow, and *bronzed diabetes*, associated with HAEMOCHROMATOSIS.
Diagnosis	The art and science of identifying a patient's disease, a prerequisite to treatment. Some diagnostic techniques date back to the time of Hippocrates: the patient's history, symptoms, and physical signs; tapping and listening, feeling, inspecting, applying all the senses. Modern tools project the perceptions of physicians into chemical and electrical processes of the body. Instruments amplify and transcribe minute currents of the heart and brain and muscles; instruments of many kinds carry trained eyes into caverns of the body; a film of tissue yields secrets to a pathologist; X-rays probe hidden structures.
Dialysis	Separation of substances in solution by passing them through a porous membrane; this is done naturally by the kidney and

mechanically by an ARTIFICIAL KIDNEY.

The transverse, dome-shaped muscle which separates the chest from the abdomen; the chief muscle of breathing. Contraction of the diaphragm expands the rib cage and lungs so that air flows in; relaxation allows the rib cage and lungs to collapse partially, and air is exhaled. A *vaginal diaphragm* is a ringed latex cup which covers the cervix for contraceptive purposes.	**Diaphragm**
See HIATUS HERNIA.	**Diaphragmatic hernia**
Abnormal frequency and liquidity of stools. In young infants, profuse diarrhoea (and vomiting) can cause serious loss of fluids and ELECTROLYTES, and the baby should be under the care of a doctor.	**Diarrhoea**
The resting stage of the heart during which relaxed chambers are filling with blood. Diastolic pressure is the lower of the two figures (such as 120/80) by which doctors express blood pressure readings (see SYSTOLE). Diastolic pressure gives the doctor significant information about the condition of blood vessels and the harmful effects of sustained hypertension.	**Diastole**
Generation of heat in body tissues by passing high-frequency electric currents through them. Resistance of the tissues produces the heat, which is very penetrating and can build up to dangerous levels unless treatment is supervised by an experienced operator. In surgical diathermy, heat is sufficient to destroy tissues or to cut tissues with little or no bleeding.	**Diathermy**
Inborn constitutional susceptibility or predisposition to a certain disease or condition.	**Diathesis**
A drug derived from the foxglove which is a powerful stimulant of heart muscle contractions. Whole digitalis contains a number of active agents called *glucosides*; some of these, such as *digitoxin*, are prepared pharmaceutically in pure form. *Digitalization* is the procedure of administering digitalis until a desired concentration of the drug is built up in the patient's body, after which maintenance doses suffice. The toxic effect of digitalis is close to the therapeutic effect and medical	**Digitalis**

	supervision of dosage is necessary.
Diopter	The unit of measurement of the refractive (light-bending) power of a lens, including the lens of the human eye, which has a power of about 10 diopters. Abbreviated as D in prescriptions for glasses; +D (plus D) indicates a convex lens for correcting a farsighted person, −D (minus D) a concave lens for correcting a short-sighted person.
Diphtheria	An acute contagious disease, once responsible for many deaths of children, but no longer a threat to the child who is properly immunized.
Diplegia	Paralysis of like parts on both sides of the body.
Diplopia	Seeing double; one object is seen as two. The condition may be temporary or persistent and can be caused by a number of diseases and disorders, including head injuries, alcoholism, and poisoning. The double vision effect is the result of paralysis or improper functioning of muscles that control the eyeball movements, or paralysis of one of the nerves controlling action of the eye muscles. Persistent double vision may be the result of a nervous system ailment such as multiple sclerosis, myasthenia gravis, meningitis, tabes dorsalis, or a brain tumour affecting the nerves running between the brain and eye muscles. Treatment of persistent diplopia may require surgery, the use of special corrective lenses, or both.
Dipsomania	Compulsion to drink alcoholic beverages to excess.
Dislocation	Displacement of a bone from its normal position in a joint, usually the result of a severe blow, fall, or twisting force; often there is an accompanying sprain.
Diuretic	An agent which increases the output of urine; a drug prescribed for this purpose. Along with other treatment, physicians prescribe diuretics for a variety of conditions associated with excessive retention of water; for example, congestive heart failure; hypertension; premenstrual tension; cirrhosis of the liver.
Diverticula	Small thin-walled pouches opening from a hollow organ. They

can occur anywhere along the digestive tract from the oesophagus to the colon, but the most common site is the colon. A person with these little pockets has *diverticulosis* but may never know it as they may not cause symptoms. It is estimated that ten per cent of people over 40 years of age have diverticulosis. Chances that existing pockets may become infected, inflamed, or ruptured, resulting in *diverticulitis*, increase with advancing age. Diverticulitis is sometimes called left-sided appendicitis because the patient's symptoms are similar to those of appendicitis except for reversal of position. Many patients with diverticulitis are well controlled with medical measures. Sometimes surgery is necessary to remove a diseased portion of the bowel.

Dizygotic

Developed at the same time from two fertilized eggs; (of twins) fraternal.

Dizziness

A feeling of unsteadiness and of the world revolving about one. The disturbance may be primarily in the inner ear, in nerves serving this area, in reduced blood supply to the brain, in nervous messages from the heart, eyes, or stomach, or in association with many other conditions. An ordinary mild bout of dizziness can usually be cured by sitting or lying down. Dizziness is not usually a symptom of serious disease but recurrent attacks should be investigated to determine the cause.

Dominant eye

The eye unconsciously preferred in visual tasks, such as aiming a rifle.

Dorsum

The back; any part of the body corresponding to the back, as the back of the hand.

Double-blind study

A technique often used in studying the effects of drugs. Neither the doctor nor the patient knows whether a given medicine contains an active drug or totally inert ingredients. This eliminates unconscious bias in knowing that a drug should not have some effect.

Double vision

See DIPLOPIA.

D

Douche	A stream of water directed against or into a part of the body; used alone, the word usually refers to a *vaginal douche*.
Down's syndrome	See MONGOLISM.
Dreams	See SLEEP.
Dropsy	An old term for OEDEMA.
Drug addiction	Certain drugs (including alcohol) have an effect on body cells, particularly those of the nervous system, called *tissue tolerance*. Body chemistry is upset and the cells adjust their metabolism to accommodate the drug. The tissues become physically dependent upon the drug to maintain their normal functions. Over a period of time, increasingly large doses of the drug are necessary to obtain the same original effect and the body, in turn, constantly alters its chemistry to accommodate the larger doses. Eventually the addict is able to tolerate doses of drugs which would be fatal to a non-addict. When an addict suddenly stops using drugs, he experiences severe WITH-DRAWAL SYMPTOMS because of physical dependency; he also has psychological dependency. Because addiction and habituation are often used interchangeably, the World Health Organization to banish confusion has adopted a more general term, drug dependence. Dependence is defined as 'a state arising from repeated administration of a drug on a periodic or continuous basis.' This is subdivided into dependence of the morphine type, cocaine type, barbiturate type, marijuana type, amphetamine type, and alcohol type, applying to all types of drug abuse.
Dry labour	See BAG OF WATERS.
Dry socket	Failure of a protective blood clot to develop in the socket left after extraction of a tooth, or premature loss of a clot, causing pain and delay in healing.
Ductus arteriosus	In the fetus, a tube which bypasses blood from the pulmonary artery to the aorta; normally it closes and ceases to function at birth. In certain cases the channel fails to close. Usually the

condition can be corrected by surgery.

Symptoms of abdominal distension, diarrhoea, vomiting, and distress, occurring soon after eating in persons whose stomachs have been partially removed.	**Dumping syndrome**
The first part of the small intestine. Here, just beyond the acid stomach, the intestinal environment begins to become alkaline. Alkaline bile and digestive juices of the pancreas flow into the duodenum. *Duodenal ulcer* is the most common type of peptic ulcer.	**Duodenum**
Thickening of connective tissue (FASCIA) of the palm of the hand, pulling one or more fingers down into the palm.	**Dupuytren's contracture**
The outermost membrane of tough connective tissue which covers the brain and spinal cord.	**Dura mater**
Abnormal state, especially of the blood.	**Dyscrasia**
Inflammation of the colon with severe diarrhoea, abdominal cramps, painful and ineffectual rectal straining; the stools may contain blood and mucus. Chemical poisons and various irritants of the bowel can cause dysentery, but there are two major forms of the disorder: BACILLARY DYSENTERY produced by certain bacteria and amoebic dysentery produced by protozoa.	**Dysentery**
Abnormality or impairment of the normal activities of an organ or bodily process.	**Dysfunction**
Literally and in its widest sense the word means difficulty in reading. This may be due to many causes, for example defective vision, mental backwardness, psychological causes, or the effects of physical disease. The word is also used to describe a particular disorder; a congenital defect of brain function, in an otherwise normal and intelligent person, which impairs or prevents his learning to read. In children, special teaching can often improve the condition.	**Dyslexia**
Impairment of speech.	**Dyslogia**

Dysmenorrhoea	Difficult, painful menstruation.
Dyspareunia	Painful or difficult sexual intercourse; the cause may be physical, mental, or both.
Dyspepsia	Disturbed digestion; indigestion. There are several disorders (see MALABSORPTION SYNDROME) in which foods are inadequately digested or assimilated. But the terms dyspepsia and indigestion are often rather casually applied to symptoms which do not arise primarily from incomplete digestion of food but which originate in the digestive canal or adjacent organs. Inaccurate use of the word does no harm if it sends one to a doctor to find out what the trouble is.
Dyspnoea	Difficult breathing, distress, often but not invariably associated with heart or lung disease.
Dystocia	Painful or difficult labour, delivery, childbirth.
Dystrophy	Degeneration, wasting, abnormal development.
Dysuria	Difficult or painful urination.

Bleeding into the skin and the discoloration of skin so produced. It may be from a bruise, or from disease of blood vessels or the blood itself.	**Ecchymosis**
An electrocardiogram. See ELECTROCARDIOGRAPH.	**ECG**
Multiple fluid-filled cysts, particularly in the liver or lungs, produced by tapeworm larvae; *hydatid disease*.	**Echinococcus cysts**
The initials mean Enteric Cytopathic Human Orphan, the orphan indicating that the viruses are not associated with known diseases. The designation has become less appropriate since some of the viruses have been identified as the causative agents of certain diseases.	**ECHO viruses**
Convulsions. A serious form which can occur in late pregnancy or even during or after delivery; it is an extreme manifestation of *toxaemia of pregnancy*, often associated with kidney disorders. Early signs of impending eclampsia are practically always evident to the doctor, in time to institute preventive measures. Eclampsia is rare in women who receive proper prenatal care.	**Eclampsia**
See SOMATOTYPE.	**Ectomorph**
In the wrong position, out of place; for example, *ectopic pregnancy* in which the embryo is implanted in a fallopian tube or elsewhere outside the uterus.	**Ectopic**
Outward-turning of an eyelid, drooping away from the eyeball.	**Ectropion**
Is not a disease, but a general term for inflammation of the skin.	**Eczema**
Toothless.	**Edentulous**
An electroencephalogram; a brain wave tracing or record. See ELECTROENCEPHALOGRAPH.	**EEG**

Effleurage	A stroking movement used in massage.
Effusion	Outpouring of fluid into a body part or tissue.
Ejaculation	Ejection of semen.
Elective treatment	Treatment which is not immediately urgent. *Elective surgery* can be put off until a more convenient or desirable time.
Electric knife	A surgical instrument employing electric current to cut and seal vessels bloodlessly.
Electrocardiograph	An instrument which amplifies tiny electric currents in contracting heart muscle and records these on paper. The written record is an *electrocardiogram* (ECG). Electric impulses are conveyed to the machine from surfaces over several areas of the heart. Interpretation of electrical events within the heart muscle, recorded in an ECG, gives valuable information in the diagnosis of heart disease and in following the progress of a patient during his recovery from a coronary attack.
Electroconvulsive therapy	(ECT) A treatment for some forms of mental illness; an electric current is passed from temple to temple through the patient's brain, producing unconsciousness. The patient has no memory of the shock.
Electroencephalograph	An instrument which amplifies minute electric currents from brain cells and transcribes them to a moving strip of paper. This record, called an *Electroencephalogram* (EEG), shows aspects of brain activity, popularly called brain waves, in the form of spiked or wavy lines. Electrodes taped to the subject's scalp pick up tiny currents from brain cells near the surface of the skull. The brain has several characteristic rhythms. Modern electroencephalographs have a number of channels, each recording changes in electric potential between two electrodes taped to different areas of the scalp. The instrument is useful in diagnosing various disturbances of brain function, such as epilepsy, and is a research tool for investigating the workings of the brain. Recent advances in studies of SLEEP and dreams have been greatly aided by the electroencephalograph's ability

to identify rhythms characteristic of different and changing levels of consciousness.

Permanent removal of superfluous hair by means of an electric needle which renders the hair follicle incapable of further growth. The word also means decomposition of a salt or chemical compound by means of an electric current.

Electrolysis

Electrolytes are dissolved salts or ions in body fluids, analogous to electrolytes in a car battery. Our electrolytes conduct electric currents, they participate in countless chemical processes of life, they are bearers of electrical energy within our cells, they are in constant motion and exert outward pressure, and they are vital regulators of acid-base balance. The principal regulator of water and electrolyte balance is the kidney. The major electrolytes are ions of sodium, chlorine, and potassium. Numerous conditions affect the composition of the body fluids: vomiting, diarrhoea, kidney or liver disease, congestive heart failure, dehydration, severe burns, diabetes, drug treatments, surgery, or oedema. There may be excessive loss or excessive retention of electrolytes. Sodium chloride (salt) locks considerable amounts of water in the body. This is the reason for *low-sodium diets*, designed to ease waterlogged tissues of their burden. But a gross deficiency of sodium may produce leg cramps and other symptoms. Correction of electrolyte deficits or excesses is an important part of the management of many illnesses.

Electrolytes

Tracings of electric currents produced by muscle action.

Electromyography

Gross enlargement of a body part (legs, scrotum) due to fluids in tissue spaces under the skin, damned back by obstruction of lymphatic drainage channels. See LYMPHOEDEMA. The most extreme forms of elephantiasis are seen in persons in tropical countries who suffer from FILARIASIS.

Elephantiasis

Menus which start with a few foods that rarely cause allergic reactions, and then add one new food at a time to determine to which one a patient reacts.

Elimination diets

Embolism	Obstruction of a blood vessel by an EMBOLUS. Consequences vary according to the size of the blocked vessel and the part of the body deprived of blood. The lungs, brain, and heart are frequent sites of embolism. *Pulmonary embolism* which can cause sudden death results from blockage of the pulmonary artery or its large branches. *Fat embolism* results from a severe injury of bone or fatty tissue which disperses fat into the bloodstream, whence it is disseminated to many organs. Fat embolism may be fatal.
Embolus	Any abnormal substance – a blood clot, fat globule, air bubble, clump of cells – which is swept along in the bloodstream until it lodges in a vessel and blocks the flow of blood.
Embryo	A term given to the developing human being in the uterus up to the third month of pregnancy, after which it is known as a fetus.
Emetic	Productive of vomiting.
Emphysema	Too much air in the lung, either from distension or, more usually, from destruction by disease of the divisions between the air sacs.
Empyema	Accumulation of pus in a body cavity, especially in the pleural cavity.
Encephalitis	Inflammation of the brain. Some forms of encephalitis are caused by viruses, others are complications of other diseases or conditions.
Encephalogram	An X-ray of the brain.
Endarterectomy	Surgical removal of a clot or plaque from the inner wall of an artery.
Endarteritis	Inflammation of the innermost layer of an artery.
Endemic	Of or relating to diseases which occur constantly or repeatedly in the same locality.

Inflammation of the lining of the heart, especially attacking the heart valves.	**Endocarditis**
Ductless glands which secrete hormones directly into the circulation.	**Endocrine glands**
A branch of dentistry concerned with disease and treatment of inner structures of the teeth.	**Endodontics**
Originating within or inside the cells or tissues.	**Endogenous**
Presence in abnormal locations of fragments of the membrane which lines the cavity of the uterus. The displaced tissue menstruates wherever situated, and so produce cystic collections of blood.	**Endometriosis**
See SOMATOTYPE.	**Endomorph**
Visual examination of hollow parts of the body by insertion of a lighted instrument through a natural outlet. There are many types (sigmoidoscope, bronchoscope, cystoscope, and others) named after the inspected organs. Some have systems of lenses, and auxiliary devices for removing foreign objects or pieces of tissue for examination.	**Endoscopy**
A toxin produced by internal processes of a germ, liberated when the cell of the germ is destroyed.	**Endotoxin**
A coating of drug tablets which permits them to pass through the acid stomach without dissolving and to liberate their dose in the alkaline intestine.	**Enteric coating**
Inflammation of the intestine, particularly of the small intestine.	**Enteritis**
Threadworm infection.	**Enterobiasis**
Viruses, such as polio and ECHO viruses, whose preferred habitat is the intestinal tract.	**Enteroviruses**

E

Enucleation	Removal of the tonsil or eyeball.
Enuresis	Bedwetting; involuntary discharge of urine.
Eosinophils	Certain white blood cells which take up a pink stain eosin. Large numbers of eosinophils are present in nasal and other secretions during allergic attacks. They are increased in parasitic infestation.
Epidemic	Rapid spread of disease attacking large numbers of people in the same locality at the same time.
Epidemic pleurodynia	See BORNHOLM DISEASE.
Epidemiology	The study of epidemic diseases.
Epidermis	Popularly, the skin; technically, the outermost part of the skin consisting of four layers without blood vessels.
Epididymitis	Inflammation of that part of the semen-conducting duct which lies upon and behind the testicle.
Epigastrium	The upper middle abdomen. A hand stretched across the lower end of the breastbone covers the epigastrium.
Epiglottis	A structure like a hinged lid above the voice box (larynx); it opens to admit air and shuts like a trapdoor during swallowing to prevent food from going down the windpipe.
Epilation	Removal of hair, including the roots. The same as DEPILATION. See ELECTROLYSIS.
Epilepsy	A nervous disorder of varying severity, marked by recurring explosive discharge of electrical activity of brain cells, producing convulsions, loss of consciousness, or brief clouding of consciousness.
Epiphysis	The end part of a long bone which in children is separated from the shaft of the bone by a layer of cartilage. It is the site of growth in long bones. As growth progresses, the cartilage

layer disappears, the epiphysis is said to have closed, and the bone does not grow longer. Therefore growth in height ceases.

An incision in the margin of the vulva to enlarge the area through which the baby's head passes in childbirth; the purpose is to prevent or minimize tearing in less desirable sites.	**Episiotomy**
A malformation of the penis in which the urinary canal remains open on the upper side of the organ. The problem is to restore urinary control and then to form a new tube by plastic surgery.	**Epispadias**
Refers to those cells that form the outer layer of the skin, those that line all the portions of the body that have contact with external air (such as the eyes, ears, nose, throat, lungs), and the liver, kidneys, digestive, urinary and reproductive tracts.	**Epithelial**
Skin tumours of varying malignancy.	**Epitheliomas**
Specialized tissue which covers all free surface of the body, forms the EPIDERMIS, lines hollow organs, glands, and respiratory passages; it does not possess blood vessels.	**Epithelium**
Epidemic disease in animals.	**Epizootic**
The name of a person applied to a disease, syndrome, or theory which it is presumed he was the first to discover or describe, for example, *Bright's disease, Addison's disease.* This form of commemoration has become less common since more precise and specific descriptions of disease have been made possible by scientific advances.	**Eponym**
A form of clubfoot.	**Equinovarus**
Poisoning with *ergot*, a substance contained in a fungus that grows on rye and other grains. Ergot has a powerful constrictive action on small blood vessels; chronic poisoning may produce closure of blood vessels, resulting in gangrene of the extremities. Various ergot drugs and combinations have medi-	**Ergotism**

cal uses, as in obstetrics and prevention of migraine headaches.

Eructation	A belch.
Erysipelas	An acute bacterial infection of the skin and underlying tissue.
Erythema	Abnormal redness of the skin. The pattern, intensity, distribution, duration, and appearance of the reddened areas give clues to disease, which may be trifling, or a disease of childhood manifested by a rash, or an allergy or systemic disorder.
Erythroblastosis (*Rh disease*)	A disease of newborn infants associated with incompatible Rh blood factors of mother and child.
Erythrocytes	Red blood cells; minute elastic discs containing HAEMOGLOBIN.
Erythrocytosis	A condition of too many red blood cells in the circulation; *polycythaemia*.
Erythropoiesis	The process of red blood cell formation.
Eschar	Sloughed-off tissue produced by a burn or corrosive substance.
Ethmoid	A bone of the upper nose behind the frontal sinus; nerve fibres of the sense of smell pass through perforations in it.
Eunuch	A castrated male; a boy or man whose testicles have been removed. Eunuchs cannot produce SPERMATOZOA or father children, but if only the testes are removed, and this operation is done after sexual maturity, some eunuchs retain a degree of sexual potency. *Eunuchoidism* is a natural condition in which the sex organs are malformed or physiologically inactive.
Euphoria	Feeling of wellbeing; often implies exaggerated elation.
Eustachian tube	A tubular passage about an inch and a half long which leads

from the middle ear to the throat. Air passing through it equalizes pressure on both sides of the eardrum, enabling the drum to vibrate freely. Infectious material can enter the middle ear through the tube.

A skin eruption or the disease which causes it. *Exanthem subitum* (also called *roseola infantum*) is a disease of childhood; fever comes on suddenly, persists for three or four days, then drops, a skin rash appears, and the child is well. The rash of scarlet fever or measles is an exanthem.	**Exanthem**
Replacement of a baby's blood with suitable whole blood of a donor; resorted to in some instances to save the life of a baby with severe blood destroying anaemia resulting from incompatibility of the mother's and baby's Rh blood factors.	**Exchange transfusion**
The act of cutting out.	**Excision**
A scratch mark of the skin, usually deep enough to bleed or become crust-covered, produced by scraping or scratching.	**Excoriation**
Peeling or shedding or surface skin in scales or sheets.	**Exfoliation**
Outpouring; glands which do not deliver their secretions to the bloodstream but through ducts and channels to organs and surfaces; for example, sweat glands, sebaceous glands, digestive glands. Inherited disabilities of the exocrine glands are the fundamental defects in CYSTIC FIBROSIS.	**Exocrine**
Originating from outside the cells or tissues.	**Exogenous**
Bulging eyes, a condition characteristic of some kinds of thyroid disease.	**Exophthalmos**
Projection of a bony growth from the surface of a bone; a bony spur.	**Exostosis**
A substance that softens or increases bronchial secretions and helps to bring up phlegm from the chest.	**Expectorant**

Exstrophy of the bladder	A congenital malformation in which the bladder has no abdominal covering and urine comes out onto the surface of the body.
Extensor	A muscle which straightens or extends a body part.
External cardiac massage	A first-aid measure to make a stopped heart start to beat, used in conjunction with mouth-to-mouth resuscitation; the latter supplies fresh oxygen. With the victim on his back, place the heel of one hand on the lower part of his breastbone (over the heart), and the other hand on top of the first one. Press down with your weight on the breastbone to force blood out of the heart into vessels. Relax the pressure; blood flows into the heart chambers. Repeat at intervals of about one second. Too much pressure can hurt the heart or break ribs; if the patient is a child, pressure of one hand may be sufficient. Ideally, one person gives mouth-to-mouth resuscitation while the other applies external heart massage. If one person must do it all, he can give external massage for half a minute, then mouth-to-mouth breathing for ten seconds or so, and repeat.
Extrasystole	A premature beat of the heart; a contraction that is triggered too soon and is followed by a compensating delay in the next beat. The pause between the premature beat and the succeeding one, which is likely to come with a thump, gives a feeling that the heart has skipped a beat. The phenomenon is quite common and usually not serious.
Extravasation	Escape of fluids from a vessel, especially a blood vessel, into surrounding tissues. A black eye is a good example.
Extrinsic asthma	A form of asthma in which the provoking substance enters the body from outside. *Intrinsic asthma*, which has its source within the body, can coexist with extrinsic asthma.
Extrinsic factor	Literally, a constituent from outside; medically, the term commonly refers to vitamin B_{12} which prevents pernicious anaemia. The vitamin is assimilated from food in conjunction with a substance secreted by the stomach called INTRINSIC FACTOR.

Anything that is exuded, oozed, trickled, pushed out. One exudes sweat, for example. Although many exudates are entirely normal, in medical usage the word often refers to pus or other materials of pathological importance.	**Exudate**
See CORNEAL TRANSPLANT.	**Eye bank**
A canine tooth	**Eye tooth**
A simple and effective eye wash can be made by adding a level teaspoon of salt to a pint of boiled water.	**Eye wash**

An operation to remove wrinkling caused by loose skin and to tighten fatty tissues which tend to sag in the face and neck with advancing years.	**Face lift**

Appearance of the face of the fetus at the outlet of the uterus during delivery, instead of the top of the head, as is normal. **Face presentation**

Contents of a bowel movement; the stool. Faeces are not simply unabsorbed food residues. The greatest part of the solid matter is made up of materials excreted from blood, and cells shed by lining membranes of the intestines; about ten per cent is bacteria (see INTESTINAL FLORA). Practically all the protein, fat, and carbohydrate that is eaten is absorbed. Unabsorbed food residues consist largely of indigestible vegetable cellulose, the amount of which varies with the diet. This indigestible roughage stimulates activity and secretions of the bowel. Large amounts of undigested food elements in faeces are associated with diseases which impair assimilation. **Faeces**

The thermometer scale formerly generally used. It marks the freezing point of water at 32 degrees F and the boiling point at 212 degrees F. See CENTIGRADE. **Fahrenheit (F)**

Brief loss of consciousness due to diminished blood supply to the brain. Usually selfcorrected; the fainting person drops to the floor and blood flows more easily to the brain. Blood vessels in the abdominal area have immense capacity to hold blood when fully dilated. Shock or strong emotion may cause these vessels to dilate and fill with so much blood that blood pressure drops and fainting results. Rarely is fainting due to heart trouble. A soldier standing at attention for some time may faint, because of lack of muscular movement to aid the return flow of blood through the veins. Feelings of faintness may be cured by lying down, or placing the head between the knees. **Fainting** (*syncope*)

Prolapse of the uterus; sagging of the organ into the lower vagina or occasionally protrusion, due to weakness, stretching, or tearing of supporting structures. **Fallen womb**

Fallopian tubes

The tubes through which the egg cell is transported to the uterus, and in which fertilization usually occurs.

Fallout

RADIOISOTOPES from nuclear explosions which settle out of the atmosphere.

False pregnancy (*pseudocyesis*)

Signs and symptoms of pregnancy occurring without conception. The woman herself is usually deceived, and even an obstetrician may be deceived for a while. The patient is usually a woman with an overpowering, obsessive desire to have a child, who through autosuggestion is somehow able to mimic the signs of pregnancy – cessation of menstruation, breast changes, morning sickness, enlargement of the abdomen at the rate of normal pregnancy. Careful examination and tests can determine that no pregnancy exists, but in some instances it is difficult to convince the woman until the expected date of delivery passes.

Fanconi's syndrome

Multiple inherited abnormalities which impair kidney function and progressively depress blood cell formation in the bone marrow.

Farmer's lung

An inflammatory disease of the lungs which principally affects agricultural workers exposed to mouldy hay, grain, fodder, or silage. The disease resembles pneumonia but does not respond to antibiotics as bacterial pneumonias do. Symptoms of chills, fever, cough, headache, and chest tightness are thought to be caused by allergy-like sensitivity to inhaled mould dusts, and may appear a few hours after heavy exposure. Total avoidance of mouldy vegetable matter is most important during the illness and after recovery.

Fascia

Tough sheets of connective tissue which give support under the skin, between and around muscles, blood vessels, nerves, and internal organs.

Fat embolism

Plugging of a blood vessel by fat droplets carried in the bloodstream; this can occur from crushing injuries of fatty tissue or bone, or injection of oily solutions.

A compound of carbon, hydrogen, and oxygen which combines with glycerol to make a fat.	**Fatty acid**
Acute anaemia with red blood cell destruction, caused by eating fava beans. The condition occurs only in genetically susceptible persons who do not possess an enzyme that is important in red blood cell metabolism. Certain drugs, such as aspirin and sulphonamides, may produce the same symptoms in susceptible persons.	**Favism**
Feverish.	**Febrile**
Chronic arthritis of rheumatoid type with enlargement of the spleen and decreased numbers of certain white blood cells.	**Felty's syndrome**
Two glands with ducts just inside the opening of the female urethra. Inflammation of the glands may involve the bladder and cause urgency of urination; the most common cause is gonorrhoeal infection.	**Female urethral glands**
The thighbone.	**Femur**
An opening in a part of the body, or the act of making one. The *fenestration operation* for improving the hearing of persons with OTOSCLEROSIS creates a bony window for passage of sound waves to the inner ear.	**Fenestration**
The period of about one week around the midpoint of the menstrual cycle when conception can occur. The fertile period cannot be pinpointed precisely, but occurs approximately from days eleven to eighteen counting from the onset of menstruation.	**Fertile period**
The taking of hurried short steps to prevent falling forwards, characteristic of *Parkinson's disease*.	**Festination**
The unborn child after the third month of pregnancy; before that it is called an embryo.	**Fetus**
Abnormally high body temperature. Normally, body tempera-	**Fever**

ture varies slightly through the day, is higher in the evening than in the morning, higher internally than at the skin surface, and is increased by eating and exercise. The most common fevers accompany infections, but disturbances of heat-regulating centres of the brain, as in heatstroke, and other noninfectious conditions can produce fever. Experienced people can often recognize fever by the feel and appearance of the patient's hot, dry, flushed skin. Accurate fever reading, however, requires the use of a thermometer. Temperature charts are kept in hospital, and may be desired by the doctor for patients under home nursing care. *Fever* increases the body's rate of metabolism about seven per cent for each degree Fahrenheit of temperature elevation. The heart's ability to contract decreases and it beats more rapidly in an attempt to move more blood to the skin to increase heat loss. Excessively high (*hyperthermic*) fever of 40.5°C (105°F) and more cannot be endured for a long period; the very high fever of HEAT-STROKE is so quickly lethal that immediate efforts to bring it down must be made by immersing the patient in an ice bath or applying a stream of cold water to the body. Young children react to the slightest infection with fever, sometimes as high as 40°C (104°F); the height of the fever does not necessarily indicate the seriousness of the infection. If a doctor cannot be reached promptly, a very high fever can be reduced by a cool sponge or cool enema. Whether or not fever is part of nature's treatment to cure infection is an unsettled question. In tissue cultures, temperatures of feverish degree inhibit the multiplication of some viruses. There is some evidence that fever increases the production of INTERFERON. But fever-producing organisms in patients survive the temperatures they produce and many authorities doubt that fever has any direct effect on the patient's resistance to infection. All agree, however, that fever is an important guide to the progress of an illness; sometimes it is the only important diagnostic clue.

Fibrillation

Fine twitching of muscle fibres, especially of the heart muscle. Individual muscle fibres act independently, uncoordinated, out of rhythm, causing rapid, irregular, ineffective heartbeats. The condition may affect the *atria* or *ventricles* of the heart. Defibrillating devices that administer an electric shock are used to restore normal rhythm.

A protein manufactured in the liver and distributed into the bloodstream where it acts as a clotting agent when a blood vessel is cut or injured. Fibrinogen combines with another substance, *thrombin*, to yield long threads of *fibrin* which form a mesh to trap blood corpuscles in a clot.	**Fibrinogen**
A muscle and connective tissue tumour of the uterus.	**Fibroid**
Inflammation of connective tissue; often, combined inflammation of muscle and connective tissue (*fibromyositis*), producing pain, tenderness, and stiffness.	**Fibrositis**
The slender bone on the outer side of the lower leg.	**Fibula**
The chronic disease caused by the presence of threadlike worms (*filaria*) in the body. The organisms get into the blood through the bites of mosquitoes. The adult worms live in the lymphatic system and cause overgrowth of fibrous tissue which obstructs drainage. Obstructed fluids accumulate in tissue spaces and cause the affected part to swell (LYMPHOEDEMA). The result is some degree of ELEPHANTIASIS. The most extreme forms of the disease occur in residents of tropical countries who are frequently reinfected from mosquito bites.	**Filariasis**
A fringelike structure; especially, fimbriae of the opening of the FALLOPIAN TUBES, close to the ovary. The fringelike projections are covered with *cilia*, minute hairlike processes which wave back and forth and set up rhythmic currents in surrounding peritoneal fluid. Their function is to sweep a mature egg cell released by the ovary into the tube where fertilization usually occurs.	**Fimbria**
See ICHTHYOSIS.	**Fish skin disease**
A break or crack in the skin or in a membrane, most frequent in the rectal area.	**Fissure**

Fistula

An abnormal channel between body parts, or leading from a hollow organ to a free surface, which usually discharges fluids or material from an organ. A fistula maybe caused by disease, injury, or an abscess which makes an abnormal drainage channel for itself. Many fistulas are named after the body parts they connect; for example, *vesicovaginal* fistula (bladder and vagina). Some fistulas never heal by themselves because of continual infection, and surgical correction is necessary to close the abnormal channels.

Flank

The fleshy outer part of the body between the ribs and hip.

Flat foot

Ordinarily, if a print of a bare foot on a piece of paper shows the sole has made flat contact all over, without an open space under the middle inside part of the foot, it is construed as a sign of flat feet caused by fallen arches. This is not always true. Babies' feet are always flat. Some people have naturally flat feet which are perfectly efficient and comfortable. When feet become *flattened*, and hurt, troubles arise and treatment is necessary.

Flatulence

Excessive gas in the stomach or intestines. A normal bowel always contains some gas; balance is maintained by unostentatious gas exchange mechanisms. Excessive gassiness, vented by belching or passing wind, may result from indiscretions of diet or some disorder of the digestive tract which requires the attention of a doctor. Sometimes, excessive belching is a consequence of unconscious AIR SWALLOWING.

Flexor

A muscle which bends a limb or part, as in flexing the biceps.

Floaters

Cells or strands of tissue which float in the VITREOUS HUMOUR and move with movements of the eyeball, casting shadows on the retina. The floaters, particularly when seen against a bright background such as open sky, look like moving spots and threads of diverse shapes. Floaters are most prevalent in nearsighted and older persons. Usually they are more annoying than serious, but if they become worrying or excessive, an eye examination is indicated.

A kidney which is abnormally movable from its normal location because of slack attachments and inadequate support from surrounding fat.	**Floating kidney**

Bacteria and other small organisms found in the intestinal contents.	**Flora (intestinal)**

Parasitic flatworms, rarely encountered, which cause infestations of the intestines, liver, or lungs.	**Flukes**

Salts of fluorine, a gaseous element. The role of fluorides in helping to lessen tooth decay is well known. Recent studies have furnished evidence that fluorides contribute importantly to normal bones as well as teeth and may play a part in the treatment and prevention of *osteoporosis*, a condition of abnormal porousness, thinning, and easy fracturing of bone, common in women after the menopause and in old people. One study of more than a thousand persons over 45 years of age has shown osteoporosis to be much less frequent in those who lived most of their lives in areas of releatively high fluoride content of drinking water than in those who lived in low-fluoride areas. There was also much less hardening of the AORTA in those who lived in high-fluoride areas. It appears that fluoride helps to keep calcium deposited in hard tissues of the body and not in soft tissues. If such action is confirmed, fluorides may assume an important preventive role in osteoporosis and hardening of the arteries.

Fluorides

A device for viewing X-ray images on a fluorescent screen. The patient stands behind the screen, and X-rays passing through the body make structures visible to the radiologist. The digestive tract, heart, lungs, and other organs can be viewed in action, and the progress of a BARIUM MEAL can be followed through the digestive tract. Closed circuit television is now used, which exposes the patient to less radiation.

Fluoroscope

Rapid, fluttery, but rhythmic beats of the heart atria.	**Flutter**

A tube inserted through the urethra into the bladder for drainage of urine; it has a small balloon at the bladder end	**Foley catheter**

which is inflated after insertion and serves to hold the catheter in place.

Folic acid

A vitamin of the B complex. Also known as *pteroylglutamic acid*. It is a bright yellow compound needed in very small amounts in the diet of animals and man. A deficiency results in poor growth, anaemia, and other blood-related disorders.

Folie à deux

A form of mental disorder, usually occurring in close friends, where both have the same delusions.

Follicle

A small sac or cavity which produces secretions or excretions. Hair grows from a follicle linked with sebaceous glands which produce skin oil.

Fontanelle

The soft spot on the top of a baby's head. The area, which is covered by a very tough membrane that is by no means so fragile as some mothers fear, will be filled with bone as the skull grows. It takes anywhere from one to two years for the spot to close.

Food diary

A complete record of everything that is eaten for a period of time, a guide to detection of food allergies.

Food poisoning

Intestinal infection caused by bacteria or their toxins in foods. Many attacks of food poisoning are not recognized for what they are. Even severe attacks with nausea, vomiting, violent diarrhoea, perhaps abdominal cramps, fever, and dizziness, may be blamed on influenza or a 24-hour virus unless several people who attended the same banquet or picnic are simultaneously stricken. The most common cause of food poisoning are strains of *salmonella* bacteria which are widespread in the animal kingdom, and *staphylococci*, readily spread by human carriers. An originally small population of salmonella in pies, eclairs, egg dishes, cakes, custards, and salads can multiply enormously if such foods are left to incubate for a short time at room temperatures. Violence of food poisoning symptoms varies with the dose of bacteria and with individual susceptibility. Attacks two or three hours after eating suggest that the poisoning was caused by bacterial toxins rather than by live bacteria. Thorough cooking destroys bacteria and some toxins (see BOTULISM) but heat must be sufficiently high, penetrating, and long continued. A large turkey may not be thoroughly cooked because the stuffing acts as a sort of intestinal insulation. Proper refrigeration and sanitation guard against food poisoning.

Drooping of the foot, due to paralysis or injury of muscles or tendons that extend or lift it.	**Foot drop**
Simple arrangements of bedding or accessories to keep the weight of blankets off a bedridden patient's upturned feet.	**Foot supports**
A perforation or opening in a body part. There are many such perforations, especially in bones, to permit passage of blood vessels and nerves. Some are abnormal, such as openings in congenitally malformed hearts.	**Foramen**
An instrument with two opposing blades and handles, for grasping, compressing, or holding body parts or surgical materials. *Forceps delivery* is extraction of the fetus from the birth canal with the mechanical aid of OBSTETRIC FORCEPS of special design.	**Forceps**
The fold of skin covering the head of the penis; the part removed in circumcision.	**Foreskin**
Sensation that ants are crawling over the skin.	**Formication**
To add one or more nutrients to a food so that it contains more of the nutrients than were present originally before processing. Milk is often fortified with vitamin D, margarine with vitamin A, beverages with vitamin C, various cereal products with thiamine and riboflavin. Foods with vitamins added to replace lost values are said to be restored.	**Fortify**
A pit or trenchlike depression in a body part.	**Fossa**
A pit, cup, or depression in a body structure; especially, the *fovea centralis*, a small depression near the centre of the retina	**Fovea**

which is the area of sharpest, most detailed vision.

Fraternal twins	Twins of either sex originating from two seperate eggs; they are no more closely related genetically than other brothers and sisters.
Free grafting	Transplantation of a completely detached piece of skin from one part of a patient's body to another.
Frenum	A fold of tissue which partially limits the movement of an organ. A small frenum can be seen as a band of tissue connecting the underside of the tongue with the floor of the mouth.
Frigidity	Sexual coldness in women. There may be some physical cause, but more often the aversion has a psychological origin which may be difficult to recognize and overcome. Frigidity which occurs after the menopause, in women who have previously had normal sex drive, may respond to hormone treatments.
Froelich's syndrome	Excessive fat deposits in the pelvic area and lack of genital development in young men, often with retardation of growth, somnolence, and other symptoms. The condition results from impairment, as by a tumour of the pituitary gland, of the functions of the *pituitary* and *hypothalamus*. Careful diagnosis is necessary because most obese, genitally underdeveloped adolescent boys do not have this specific disorder.
Frozen section	A piece of tissue removed from the body, and quickly frozen by carbon dioxide spray, sliced, and examined immediately under a microscope. This is most often done when cancer is suspected and the patient is on the operating table, while surgeons await the verdict which will determine the extent of the operation.
Frozen shoulder	Pain, stiffness, and limitation of movement in the shoulder and upper arm.
Frozen sperm	SPERMATOZOA frozen at very low temperatures, with a small amount of glycerol added, come alive when thawed and are

F

capable of fertilization. See ARTIFICIAL INSEMINATION.

Follicle-stimulating hormone.	**FSH**
Destruction of tissue by DIATHERMY.	**Fulguration**
Sudden in onset, explosive, severe, rapid in course.	**Fulminating**
Disease without any discoverable organic basis.	**Functional disease**
The part of a hollow organ farthest from its opening: for example, the back part of the eye; the top part of the uterus farthest from its cervical outlet.	**Fundus**
Forms of plant life, including moulds and yeasts, some of which are capable of causing infection. For example, *mycoses; ringworm; otitis externa; thrush; yeast infections*.	**Fungi**
A congenital deformity in which the breastbone is depressed towards the spine, forming a more or less funnel-shaped cavity. The deformity rarely affects the heart and lungs adversely unless unrelated diseases are present.	**Funnel chest** (*pectus excavatum*)
The upper end of the ulna at the elbow, so-called because a blow there causes the fingers to tingle.	**Funny bone**
A boil.	**Furuncle**
Spindle-shaped.	**Fusiform**
Union, cohesion, merging together; for example, *spinal fusion*, the uniting of two vertebrae by disease or by surgical procedures to improve some painful condition of the back. Also, the fusion of images from the two eyes for efficient binocular vision.	**Fusion**

G

An agent that promotes the flow of milk.	**Galactagogue**

A hereditary condition of infants who cannot digest milk sugars (*lactose, galactose*) because their bodies lack a necessary enzyme. Milk feedings lead to toxic accumulations of galactose in the blood, injuring the lens of the eye, the brain, and kidneys, with formation of cataracts and mental retardation unless all milk and milk products are immediately and stringently removed from the diet. The outlook with strict dietary control is good, and children who survive early infancy are often normal. Galactosaemia is inherited as a recessive trait. If a galactosaemic infant is born into a family, the doctor should test later offspring of the same parents and institute a galactose-free diet immediately after birth if necessary. — **Galactosaemia**

The saclike organ attached to the liver in which bile is stored, concentrated, and delivered to the digestive tract as needed. — **Gallbladder**

Sounds of the heart resembling the gallop of a horse, indicative of failing heart muscle. — **Gallop rhythm**

Stones in the gallbladder; they may or may not cause symptoms. — **Gallstones**

A germ cell; an egg or sperm. — **Gamete**

An IMMUNOGLOBULIN; a protein in the blood which gives immunity to certain diseases through ANTIBODY production. Gamma globulin injections containing specific antibodies are sometimes given in the hope of preventing an infection in a person who has been exposed to it, or making it milder. Antibodies which protect against bacterial and viral infections are mostly in gamma globulin circulating in the blood; other closely related immunoglobulins occur in internal and external secretions outside the blood, as in saliva, tears, nasal, bronchial, and intestinal fluids. — **Gamma globulin**

A cyst of a tendon sheath on the back of the wrist. If troublesome, it can be removed surgically. A *ganglion* is also a cluster of nerve cells which serves as a centre of nervous activity. — **Ganglion** (usually of the wrist)

Ganglionic blockage agents	Drugs, prescribed for some patients with high blood pressure, which reduce the actions of ganglia that transmit impulses which constrict blood vessels and increase pressures. Ganglionic blockers produce the greatest fall in blood pressure when the patient is standing, relatively little change when the patient is lying down. Sometimes a patient who has been lying down may feel faint when he suddenly rises to a sitting position.
Gangrene	Death of tissue due to failure of blood supply to the area. There are many precipitating causes – vascular disease, frostbite, burns, crush injury, pressure, obstruction of blood vessels, too tight a tourniquet. *Wet gangrene* has an offensive watery discharge and becomes infected so that complications of infection are superimposed upon the gangrene. Amputation of the part may be necessary to save the patient's life. *Dry gangrene* does not become infected but the part becomes dry and mummified. Small areas of dry gangrene may sometimes be saved by appropriate treatment, but amputation may be necessary. Diabetics are especially prone to gangrene of the feet and legs and preventive measures are very important.
Gargoylism	A hereditary condition in children characterized by opacities of the cornea, protruding abdomen, large head, short arms and legs, mental deficiency.
Gas gangrene	A serious infection of injured tissues with bacilli which produce bubbles of foul-smelling gas.
Gastrectomy	Surgical removal of all or part of the stomach.
Gastric analysis	Analysis of stomach juices for acidity, presence of cells, and other elements. The juice, obtained after the patient has fasted twelve hours, is withdrawn with a syringe connected to a tube passed through the nose into the stomach.
Gastric flu	A term more current among patients than doctors. Usually the complaint is of nausea, vomiting, and diarrhoea, which run their course in a couple of days or even 24 hours and have nothing to do with influenza. Gastrointestinal viruses may cause such upsets but it is practically never possible to identify

the viruses. Many cases of self-diagnosed gastric flu may actually be instances of unsuspected FOOD POISONING.

A treatment sometimes used for peptic ulcer; the patient swallows a balloon which is cooled by passing freezing agents through it.	**Gastric freezing**
Inflammation of the stomach.	**Gastritis**
The long muscle of the inner side of the lower leg which bends the leg and extends the foot.	**Gastrocnemius**
Inflammation of the stomach and intestines, producing such symptoms as diarrhoea, abdominal pain, nausea, vomiting, fever. There are many causes; infections, food poisoning, parasites, allergies, bacteria, viruses, and toxins.	**Gastroenteritis**
Joining the stomach to a loop of intestine to bypass the duodenum.	**Gastroenterostomy**
Of or relating to the stomach and intestines.	**Gastrointestinal**
A surgically created outlet of the stomach onto the skin surface of the abdomen.	**Gastrostomy**
A disorder of LIPID metabolism, transmitted as a recessive trait. It is characterized by enlarged spleen and liver, bone and joint pains, and brown pigmentation of the skin, due to accumulation of abnormal fatlike substances.	**Gaucher's disease**
Feeding of liquid nutrients into the stomach by a tube.	**Gavage**
The units involved in transmission of hereditary characteristics, contained in the CHROMOSOMES.	**Genes**
The reproductive organs.	**Genitalia**
Of or relating to genital and urinary organs – kidneys, ureters, bladder, urethra, prostate, testes – which are interrelated.	**Genitourinary**

Geographic tongue

Fancied resemblance of the surface of the tongue to a relief map gives this disorder its name. Thickened patches occur on the tongue and shift positions from day to day. This odd appearance is the only symptom. The cause is not known. The disorder usually occurs in children and adolescents; debilitated persons appear to be more susceptible.

Geophagia

Dirt-eating. See PICA.

Geotrichosis

An infection caused by species of fungi, affecting mucous membranes of the mouth, lungs, or intestinal tract. Chronic cough is a common symptom. The condition responds well to proper treatment.

Geriatrics

The medical specialty concerned with care of old people.

German measles
(*rubella*)

A mild viral infection producing a pink rash which spreads all over the body, sometimes with symptoms of headache and slight fever, sometimes with symptoms so slight that the infection passes unnoticed. On the other hand rubella in a woman in the first three months of pregnancy may cause serious damage to the embryo.

Gestation

Pregnancy.

G.I.

Gastrointestinal.

Gigantism

Abnormal tallness, most often a result of excessive secretion of GROWTH HORMONE by the pituitary gland before the growing ends of the bones have closed, but other factors may produce excessive height. Boys up to six feet are not considered to be giants; they fall at one extreme of a normal bell-shaped distribution curve of height in the population, with unusually short people who are not dwarfs at the other extreme.

Gingiva

The gum. *Gingivitis*, inflammation of the gums, is the most common form of *periodontal* disease.

Gland

A cell or organ which makes and releases hormones or other substances used in the body. *Endocrine* glands secrete their products into the bloodstream; *exocrine* glands, to body surfaces or elsewhere, by ducts or channels (for example, sweat glands).

INFECTIOUS MONONUCLEOSIS.	**Glandular fever**

A common cause of blindness in adults, produced by destructive pressure of fluid inside the eye. An acute form may come on suddenly and cause intense pain; a chronic form may cause no symptoms that the patient is aware of, although his vision is being insidiously impaired. Measurement of internal pressures of the eye with a *tonometer* is an important part of an eye examination. The condition is treated either by instillation of eye-drops, or by operation.
Glaucoma

Chronic gonorrhoeal discharge.
Gleet

Supporting cells and fibres of nervous tissue. *Glioma* is a tumour of glial tissue, occurring principally in the brain and spinal cord.
Glia

One type of protein in the blood plasma.
Globulin

A 'lump in the throat' which does not disappear on swallowing; also called *globus sensation* when no disease or organic cause can be discovered. The condition, most common in women, is associated with anxiety, and tightness or spasms of throat muscles. The feeling may also be caused by a foreign object in the throat, or swelling of lymphoid tissues such as tonsils or adenoids. The complaint, if persistent, calls for medical examination to rule out possible physical causes.
Globus

Tufted networks of capillaries which bring blood to chambers of the kidney for filtration of waste materials.
Glomeruli

Acute or chronic inflammation of fine blood vessels of the glomeruli, usually preceded by a streptococcal infection.
Glomerulonephritis

Inflammation of the tongue.
Glossitis

Glottis	The aperture between the vocal cords, including parts of the voice box concerned with sound production.
Glucagon	A hormone produced by cells of the pancreas, comparable to insulin but opposite in action. Glucagon's function is to correct LOW BLOOD SUGAR levels by stimulating the liver to convert more of its reserves of GLYCOGEN into sugar.
Glucocorticoids	Cortisone-like hormones of the adrenal gland which influence carbohydrate, protein, and fat metabolism.
Glucose tolerance test	A test for early diabetes and other metabolic disorders. It measures the patient's ability to reduce blood sugar levels at a normal rate. After fasting, a blood sugar level is taken as a baseline and the subject is given a measured amount of dissolved sugar to drink. Blood sugar levels are taken at half-hourly intervals. Abnormal rise or persistence of blood sugar is indicative of diabetes. The test is used in borderline cases.
Glue-sniffing	The dangerous and foolish practice of inhaling volatile intoxicating fumes of airplane glues and similar cements, indulged in by some teenagers.
Gluteal	Of or relating to the *gluteus* muscles of the buttocks.
Gluten-free diet	A regimen which excludes wheat, rye, oats, and their products from the diet of patients with *coeliac disease*. See MALABSORPTION SYNDROME.
Glycerol	Glycerine.
Glycogen	Animal starch, similar to vegetable starch; the form in which carbohydrate is stored in the liver and released as energy needs demand. The liver manufactures glycogen from DEXTROSE (glucose), a sugar, and reconverts glycogen to sugar as needed.
Glycogen storage disease	A group of hereditary disorders of infants. The infant lacks certain enzymes necessary for glucose metabolism. This leads

to abnormal deposits of glycogen in various tissues of the body, with progressive slowing down of body processes.

Sugar in the urine.	**Glycosuria**
Enlargement of the thyroid gland. There are several types.	**Goitre**
Substances such as are contained in plants of the cabbage family and some other vegetables, which in excessive amounts induce goitre.	**Goitrogens**
Compounds of gold, used in progressive, crippling *rheumatoid arthritis* in the hope of suppressing the active inflammatory disease and decreasing bone and cartilage destruction.	**Gold salts**
The primary sex glands, ovaries or testes.	**Gonads**
An instrument for studying angles of the eye where fluids drain.	**Gonioscope**
The most common venereal disease, an infection produced by kidney-shaped bacteria. Recovery from gonorrhoea does not give significant future immunity; reinfection is frequent. Incidence of the disease has increased in recent years.	**Gonorrhoea**
A specific form of arthritis associated with gonorrhoea, responsive to penicillin.	**Gonorrhoeal arthritis**
A serious eye disease of newborn infants, acquired in passage through the birth canal of a mother who has gonorrhoea. Obstetricians sometimes put drops into the baby's eyes at birth to prevent the infection.	**Gonorrhoeal ophthalmia**
Little skin bumps induced by cold or shock. The bumps arise around hair follicles in response to minute muscles which attempt to raise the hair.	**Gooseflesh**
A hereditary disorder of body chemistry, resulting in too much uric acid in the blood, with chalklike deposits of urate crystals (derived from uric acid) in cartilage of the joints and some-	**Gout**

times elsewhere.

GP　　　　　General practitioner.

Graafian follicles　　　Tiny, round, transparent cysts embedded in the ovary. Each follicle contains an immature egg cell. Under the influence of the follicle-stimulating hormone of pituitary gland, one of the blisters is stimulated to grow, and its egg matures in preparation for fertilization. The follicle bursts at about the fourteenth day of the menstrual cycle and releases the ripened egg; this is called *ovulation*.

Gram-positive, -negative　　　Classification of bacteria according to whether they do or do not accept a stain, named after Hans Gram, a Danish bacteriologist. Different life processes and vulnerabilities of germs are reflected by their Gram-positive or Gram-negative characteristics. For instance, an antimicrobial drug effective against certain Gram-positive germs may be ineffective against Gram-negative ones, or vice versa.

Grand mal　　　Severe epileptic seizure; convulsions, loss of consciousness, jerking and stiffening of the body.

Granulation tissue　　　Tiny red, rounded, fleshy masses having a soft granular appearance; the type of tissue that forms in early stages of wound healing. Each granule has new blood vessels and reparative cells. Proud flesh is an excessive overgrowth of granulation tissue.

Granulocytes　　　White blood cells containing granules that become conspicuous when dyed. They are manufactured in the red marrow of the bones. One of their functions is to digest and destroy invading bacteria.

Granuloma　　　A tumour, new growth, or chronically inflamed area in which GRANULATION TISSUE is prominent.

Granuloma inguinale　　　A mildly contagious venereal disease produced by rod-shaped bacteria. It is named after the *inguinal* region (groin) where lesions appear.

Fine, sandlike particles of the same substance as kidney stones, often eliminated in the urine without anything being noticed.	**Gravel**
Hyperthyroidism, toxic goitre.	**Graves's disease**
Pregnant. In obstetrician's language, a *gravida* is a pregnant woman; a *primigravida*, one who is pregnant for the first time; a *multigravida*, one who has had several pregnancies.	**Gravid**
An incomplete fracture of a long bone, usually in children whose bones are still pliable. The break does not go all the way through the bone, which is splintered on one side only, in much the same way that a green stick splinters on the outside if you hold an end in each hand and bend it until it breaks.	**Greenstick fracture**
CARTILAGE	**Gristle**
The lowest part of the abdomen where it joins the legs; the groove at this junction. Also called the *inguinal* area, a common site of a hernia.	**Groin**
Semi-fluid material which fills spaces between connective tissue fibres and cements them together.	**Ground substance**
Pain in a child's legs or arms may be associated with subacute rheumatic fever and the complaint should be investigated by a doctor, but there are other quite harmless causes of what are called growing pains. Non-rheumatic muscle pains at night are quite common in normal children. These pains are most probably an after-effect of vigorous playtime activities. They usually occur in muscles of the legs and thighs at the end of the day or soon after the child goes to sleep; there is no pain on motion and the child does not limp; he is vague in pointing out where it hurts and is free of pain in the morning. In fact, except for cutting teeth, growing is painless. So-called growing pains should always be investigated in case they are due to disease.	**Growing pains**
A hormone of the anterior pituitary gland which stimulates growth.	**Growth hormone**

G.U.	Genitourinary.
Guaiac test	A dye test, usually of urine or a stool specimen, for the presence of blood.
Gullet	The oesophagus; the muscular tube through which food passes from mouth to stomach.
Gumboil	A swelling of the gum produced by an abscess at the root of a tooth, usually painful.
Gumma	A firm, rubbery mass of tissue resembling GRANULATION TISSUE, occurring almost anywhere in the body but most frequently in the skin, heart, liver, or bones. It is a characteristic lesion of late syphilis.
Guthrie test	A blood test for *phenylketonuria*.
Gynaecoid	Resembling a woman; female-like; as, a gynaecoid pelvis.
Gynaecologist	A physician who specializes in diseases of women.
Gynaecomastia	Abnormal enlargement of either or both male breasts. It may result from therapeutic use or unintentional absorption of female hormones, from glandular abnormalities, from drugs such as digitalis, amphetamine, or reserpine, or it may be associated with conditions which have little in common, such as thyroid disease, adrenal or testicular tumours, cirrhosis of the liver. Gynaecomastia frequently occurs in perfectly healthy adolescent boys and usually disappears in a few weeks; this form is a transient phase of the body's coming into mature hormonal balance.

A red, often elevated birthmark; strawberry mark. It may or may not be present at birth. Only superficial blood vessels are involved. The mark often disappears spontaneously after some months, but in some cases treatment may be required.

Haemangioma

Vomiting of blood.

Haematemesis

A swelling produced by effusion of blood into a cavity.

Haematocele

The percentage by volume of red blood cells in whole blood; a reading is obtained by spinning whole blood in a centrifuge to pack the cells.

Haematocrit

A swelling filled with blood which clots to form a solid mass. The blood accumulates from vessels injured by a blow or disease. A *subdural haematoma* is one that occurs under the skull. The cauliflower ear of boxers results from a neglected haematoma.

Haematoma

Blood in the urine. *Occult* blood in the urine is not visible but can be detected by tests. Haematuria may occur from relatively harmless causes (for example, prolonged marching, and severe stress of physical contact sports), but it may portend serious disease and always requires medical investigation.

Haematuria

A progressive disease characterized by abnormal deposits of iron in many organs of the body, associated with bronzing of the skin, diabetes, and impaired functioning of the liver and pancreas. Mild forms of the disease with few if any clinical symptoms may require liver biopsy to make the diagnosis. It is thought that the patient has an abnormal capacity to absorb iron, rather than lessened ability to excrete it, and that the trait is genetically determined. A key treatment of severe haemochromatosis is frequent bloodletting (PHLEBOTOMY) as often as once a week, to deplete the stores of iron that harm the patient.

Haemochromatosis
(*bronzed diabetes*)

A device for counting blood cells.

Haemocytometer

Separation of waste materials from blood by passage over a

Haemodialysis

semipermeable membrane, especially as performed by an artificial kidney.

Haemoglobin	The colouring matter of red blood cells. The molecule contains a protein part (*globin*) joined with an iron-containing pigment, *haem* (from which comes the prefix *haem-* for many medical words denoting some relationship to the blood). *Haem* is the oxygen-carrying portion of haemoglobin. Haemoglobin picks up oxygen in the lungs, holds it loosely, carries it in arterial blood, and delivers it as a fuel to cells. In exchange, the blood plasma picks up carbon dioxide which cells must get rid of and carries it to the lungs where it is exhaled, while a fresh load of oxygen is taken on. Iron is the key element of this remarkable gas-transporting molecule but the protein part is vital too; not all kinds of anaemias are benefited by merely taking iron.
Haemolysis	Dissolution, breakdown of red cells with release of HAEMO- GLOBIN. Old worn-out red cells are constantly being broken down and replaced; the process balances out in healthy persons. Excessive haemolysis may result from chemicals, incompatible transfusions, snake venom, and congenital or acquired conditions leading to haemolytic jaundice and anaemia.
Haemophilia	A bleeding disease. Hope that haemophilia may be conquered received great impetus in 1967 with development of concentrated antihaemophilic globulin for preventing bleeding episodes.
Haemoptysis	Coughing up blood.
Haemorrhage	Bleeding. The only normal form of bleeding is menstruation. Otherwise, bleeding is a sign of something wrong, often the major symptom to be dealt with immediately in giving first aid. *Arterial bleeding* comes in spurts of bright red blood with each beat of the heart, unless blood wells up into a wound from a deep artery. *Venous bleeding* is indicated by a continuous flow of dark blood. *Capillary bleeding* is a general oozing from a raw surface such as a grazed knee. *Internal bleeding* is to be suspected if the patient has suffered severe blows, crushing,

falls, or penetrating injuries which may lacerate internal organs. Disease, such as erosion of a peptic ulcer, may cause haemorrhage into closed body cavities, with signs of shock.

Dilated varicose veins in and around the rectal opening. The condition is common, is often tolerated quite well for years, sometimes is temporary, as in pregnancy, and frequently responds to medical treatment and improvement of bowel habits. Haemorrhoids may shrink by themselves, or get worse. Some are best removed by surgical operation, *haemorrhoidectomy*. | **Haemorrhoids** (piles)

An instrument which stops bleeding by clamping a blood vessel, or an agent which stops bleeding. | **Haemostat**

See ALOPECIA. | **Hair transplants**

A rare condition which may occur after use of antibiotics, or from unknown causes; intertwining hairlike filaments form black or brownish patches on the tongue. The disease, if it may be called such, is harmless. The hairy patches may disappear quickly or persist for months. | **Hairy tongue**

Chemical agents which produce distortions of the mind. | **Hallucinogenic drugs**

The big toe. | **Hallux**

See BUNION. | **Hallux valgus**

A toe which is bent upwards like an inverted V and cannot flatten out, usually caused by cramping the toes into too small a shoe. | **Hammer toe**

Tendons above the back of the knee. | **Hamstrings**

An insidiously developing disease in the first decade of life, manifested by bulging eyes, excessive thirst, deposits of CHOLESTEROL in bones and tissue under the skin. | **Hand-Schuller-Christian disease**

See LEPROSY. | **Hansen's disease**

Hashimoto's disease

A form of chronic thyroiditis occurring most frequently in middle-aged women. It is thought to be an AUTO-IMMUNE DISEASE.

Hay fever

Pollinosis; an allergic reaction to inhaled pollens, characterized by reddened weepy eyes, running nose, and sneezing.

Hearing aids

Choice of the right hearing aid requires hearing tests by an ear specialist, since there are many kinds of hearing impairment, improved by different types of instruments. The ear specialist will suggest which type of hearing aid is suitable. The decision depends upon the type of hearing loss, its severity, and other factors. The specialist may suggest a National Health Service instrument or a brand-name of hearing aid. In selecting a hearing aid: Compare for clarity and quality of sound. Listen to familiar voices with different aids. Compare how well you understand speech with each of the aids. Listen in noisy places as well as in quiet. Try the aids outdoors as well as indoors. Compare for comfort and convenience. Controls should be easy to operate. Batteries, parts, and minor repairs should be available locally. Compare costs. A low-priced aid may be just as satisfactory as a high-priced aid, depending on your needs. Does the price include the ear mould, the cord and the receiver, and the battery? Ask about the costs of batteries. Compare services. Does the dealer give you a convenient repair and replacement service? Will the dealer help you to learn to use your aid?

Heart attack

Common term for *coronary thrombosis*.

Heart block

Heart block, of various degrees, occurs when the transmission of impulses from the atria to the ventricles is interfered with.

Heartburn

Mild to severe burning sensations in the upper abdomen or beneath the breastbone, usually resulting from regurgitation of stomach contents into the oesophagus. Heartburn typically occurs after a heavy meal containing fatty foods, often occurs when the patient is lying down, or sitting with feet slightly elevated, and is relieved by sitting up. Occasional heartburn associated with dietary excess is not uncommon and does not necessarily require treatment. Weight reduction, antacids, diet regulation, and sleeping with the head of the bed elevated are helpful measures. Persistent or severe heartburn, or pain thought to be heartburn, may be associated with disease requiring medical diagnosis. Heartburn is the most common symptom of *hiatus hernia*. It is frequent in the middle and later months of pregnancy.

Heart-lung machine

A device which infuses oxygen into a patient's venous blood (a lung function) and pumps the freshened blood to the circulation (a heart function). Several types of such devices make open heart surgery feasible.

Heart murmurs

Various sorts of blowing, soft, or swishing sounds made by the heart. The mere presence of murmurs does not necessarily indicate serious disease. Some murmurs are congenital, some are acquired (as from rheumatic fever), some are functional and of no great significance. Murmurs are heard in many healthy children and adults. The meaning of murmurs, as of all signs, must be interpreted by a physician.

Heat cramps

Painful muscle spasms of legs and abdomen, resulting from loss of salt through profuse prolonged sweating.

Heatstroke

A very serious reaction to exposure to extreme heat. The heat-regulating centres in the brain are paralyzed; the victim's extremely high temperature must be reduced immediately with ice packs or streams of cold water.

Heberden's nodes

Small swellings at the end joints of the fingers in older people. The condition is a form of osteoarthritis which does not progress to severe crippling. The classic description by William Heberden is as valid today as when he published his account in 1802: '. . . little hard knobs, about the size of a small pea, which are frequently seen upon the fingers, particularly a little below the top, near the joint. They have no connection with the gout, being found in persons who never had it; they continue for life; and being hardly ever attended by pain, or disposed to become sores, are rather unsightly than inconvenient, though they must be of some little hindrance to the free use of the finger."

Helminthiasis	Infestation with *helminths*, parasitic worms.
Hemianopsia	Half vision; blindness of one half of the field of vision. One or both eyes may be affected.
Hemiplegia	Paralysis of one side of the body, due to a clot or rupture of a brain artery (stroke). It may be temporary or permanent, and associated with hemianaesthesia.
Henoch-Schönlein purpura	An allergic form of haemorrhage into the skin, beginning with pain in the abdomen and joints. Recovery is usually spontaneous unless the kidneys are affected. The condition may be associated with streptococcal infection, rheumatic fever, or food allergy.
Hepatitis	Usually virus-caused inflammation of the liver. There are also nonviral forms, such as amoebic, alcoholic, toxic, and syphilitic.
Hepatolenticular degeneration	See WILSON'S DISEASE.
Hepatoma	A tumour of the liver.
Hermaphrodite	A person with the sex organs of both sexes. True hermaphrodites are rare. More common are *pseudohermaphrodites*, examples of *intersex*. Such persons, assigned to the wrong sex at birth, may in later life be candidates for sex reversal operations, which do not actually change the basic sex, but give it better expression. Assignment of true sex at birth can be very difficult because of great variation in external and internal structures. Males with HYPOSPADIAS and CRYPTORCHIDISM may be assigned a female role; females may be mistaken for males with these abnormalities. Surgical exploration is often necessary in doubtful cases, and it may be possible for surgery to correct the condition, if not completely, at least to a degree of satisfactory adjustment. But the varieties of hermaphroditism are far too numerous and complex for any

single rule of sex assignment. Even the genetic sex may be wrong. Girls with testicular feminization have internal testes and are genetically male, but they have a body of normal female appearance, with a vagina but without a uterus or menstruation; their hormones at puberty are exclusively feminizing and their entire psychological outlook is feminine. Cases of doubtful sex require individual study and technical knowledge. If the sex of an infant is in doubt, appropriate steps, surgical or otherwise, should be taken at an early age, not only that the child may identify with its appropriate sex, but because in some cases an endocrine disturbance detrimental to health may underlie the condition.

Protrusion of an organ or part of an organ through a weak spot in tissues which normally contain it. There can be herniations of the brain, lung, or other organs, but the most common herniations are of organs contained by the abdominal wall. A natural weak spot in the groin area, especially in men, who have an opening through which the spermatic cord passes, is the site of *inguinal* hernia, the most common type in both men and women. It is curable by surgical operation, as indeed are other forms of hernia.	**Hernia** (*rupture*)
Any operation for repair of hernia whch includes suturing.	**Herniorraphy**
A COXSACKIE VIRUS infection, usually of infants and children, producing fever, sore throat, loss of appetite, sometimes nausea and vomiting.	**Herpangina**
The cold sore or fever blister.	**Herpes simplex**
See SHINGLES.	**Herpes zoster**
Protrusion of part of the stomach into the chest cavity through a weak spot in the DIAPHRAGM.	**Hiatus hernia**
The annoyance is known to all; its medical definition is spasmodic contraction of the DIAPHRAGM and sudden closure of the glottis. Irritation of nerves that control the diaphragm causes spasm, and the glottis, the chink between the vocal	**Hiccups** (hiccough)

cords, snaps shut, causing a peculiar sound. The hiccup trigger may be an overloaded stomach, trapped gas, something that went down the wrong way, swallowing hot foods or irritants, gulping, or unknown trifling provocations. Virtually all the popular cures for hiccups (re-breathing from a paper bag, holding the breath as long as possible, taking a dozen sips of water without stopping to breathe) increase the carbon dioxide content of the lungs and thus help to stabilize the breathing centre. Severe hiccups which continue for hours or days may be associated with liver, abdominal, or intestinal disease, or lesions of the breathing centre; temporary surgical interruption of the phrenic nerve may be necessary to stop incessant spasms.

Hip dislocation
(congenital)

Spontaneous dislocation of the hip before or shortly after birth.

Hippocratic oath

A statement of ethics traditionally demanded of the young physician on entering practice. It contains some anachronisms – mention of freemen and slaves, and apparent ruling out of operations for bladder stone (*lithotomy*) as beneath the dignity of reputable men of medicine. But the ethical precepts of the Oath endure. The Oath bears the name of Hippocrates, the famous Greek physician, born about 460 B.C., who is called the Father of Medicine for his sound and close observations of patients and diseases which began to give the medical arts a scientific foundation, but whether or not Hippocrates himself wrote the Oath is not known; it is probably a collective expression of his followers. There are several English translations of the Oath; the wording that follows is best known: 'I swear by Apollo the physician, by Aesculapius, Hygeia, and Panacea, and I take to witness all the gods, all the goddesses, to keep according to my ability and my judgment the following Oath To consider dear to me as my parents him who taught me this art, to live in common with him and if necessary to share my goods with him, to look upon his children as my own brothers, to teach them this art if they so desire without fee or written promise, to impart to my sons and the sons of the master who taught me and the disciples who have enrolled themselves and have agreed to the rules of the profession, but to these alone, the precepts and instruction. I will prescribe regimen for the good of my patients according to my ability and my judgment and never do harm to anyone. To please no one will I give a deadly drug, nor give advice which may cause his death. Nor will I give a woman a pessary to procure abortion. But I will preserve the purity of my life and my art. I will not cut for stone, even for patients in whom the disease is manifest. I will leave this operation to be performed by specialists in this art. In every house where I come I will enter only for the good of my patients, keeping myself far from all intentional ill-doing and all seduction, and especially from the pleasures of love with women or with men, be they free or slaves. All that may come to my knowledge in the exercise of my profession or outside of my profession or in daily commerce with men, which ought not to be spread abroad, I will keep secret and will never reveal. If I keep this oath faithfully, may I enjoy my life and practise my art, respected by all men and in all times, but if I swerve from it or violate it, may the reverse be my lot."

See MEGACOLON.	**Hirschsprung's disease**
Abnormal hairiness.	**Hirsutism**
A normal chemical of body cells which plays a part in allergic reactions.	**Histamine**
Systemic infection due to inhalation of dusts containing spores of a species of fungus.	**Histoplasmosis**
Generally a trivial symptom resulting from using the voice too much; if it persists for more than a couple of weeks, a doctor should be consulted to determine the cause.	**Hoarseness**
A liver studded with small nodules, the most common form of CIRRHOSIS OF THE LIVER.	**Hobnail liver**
A form of malignancy of the lymph nodes.	**Hodgkin's disease**
Infestation of the small intestine by a parasitic worm.	**Hookworm**

Hordeolum	A stye, or abscess of the eyelid.
Horseshoe kidney	Kidneys linked at their lower ends by a band of tissue instead of being separate; their shape somewhat resembles a horseshoe.
Hot flushes	See MENOPAUSE.
Household pets	The family dog, cat, or other pet is a pleasure-giving member of the household – if the animal is healthy and well cared for. Puppies and kittens should be wormed by a vet to prevent contamination of soil and materials with worm eggs in their excretions. Ingested eggs of the common dog roundworm can enter the bloodstream and larvae can reach many parts of the body. Mysterious cases of SCABIES, the itch, have occurred in persons who never dreamed that the family dog carried the mites. Animals with fur or feathers (even stuffed toy ones) are suspect if someone in the family has allergies, even though skin tests may not show sensitivity to a particular animal. Allergic persons have a tendency to become sensitized to scurf. Pets should have veterinary attention if they show any of the following symptoms: abnormal discharges; abnormal lumps or difficulty in getting up or lying down; loss of appetite, marked weight loss or gain, or excessive water consumption; excessive head shaking, scratching, and biting any part of the body.
Housemaid's knee	Inflammation of the knee bursa.
Housewife's eczema	A dermatitis associated with soaps, detergents, and water.
Humour	Any fluid or semi-fluid of the body; for example, aqueous and vitreous humours of the eye. There is no connection with the ancient humoral theory of disease, which held that sickness results from disproportions of four body humours – blood, phlegm, yellow bile, and black bile – respectively associated with sanguine, phlegmatic, choleric, and melancholic temperaments. The word melancholy literally means black bile.
Hunner's ulcer	An ulcer of the lining of the urinary bladder, associated with chronic interstitial cystitis (shrinkage of the bladder wall,

splitting, decreased capacity).

A rare hereditary disease, appearing in middle life or later; there is progressive deterioration of the nervous system, manifested in jerky involuntary movements of the arms, legs, and face; personality changes, speech defects, difficulties of walking and swallowing. Profound nervous degeneration ultimately leads to idiocy and death. The disease is transmitted as a dominant trait. Members of families in which the disease has appeared should have the benefit of genetic counselling; if they are carriers of the defective genes, half their children, statistically, will have the disease, and for that reason they may choose to forgo parenthood.	**Huntington's chorea**

Widely spaced, narrow-edged upper central incisors with notching at the biting edge; a sign of congenital syphilis, though not always of that origin.

Hutchinson's teeth

A condition of pronounced respiratory distress which affects newborn infants, especially premature infants, at birth, and may be fatal in a day or two. It is the most common cause of death of live-born premature infants. The affected infant cannot get enough oxygen because ducts leading to tiny air sacs in the lungs are lined with hyaline (glassy) material, probably derived from the baby's own secretions. Breath is rapid and laboured almost from the moment of birth; CYANOSIS appears; the heart works desperately to push enough blood through the lungs. Absence of a substance, surfactant, which reduces surface tension and normally lines the air sacs seems to be the most important abnormality. Treatment consists of measures to avoid premature delivery if possible, rapid resuscitation at birth of premature infants, care in an incubator and, recently, the forcing of moist oxygen-rich air under pressure into the infant's lungs.

Hyaline membrane disease

Infestation with animal tapeworms which produce clusters of fluid-filled cysts in the lungs and other organs.

Hydatid disease

A rare complication of early pregnancy, resulting from degeneration of membranes which would normally become a part of

Hydatidiform mole

the placenta. The mass resembles a bunch of grapes of irregular size.

Hydramnios	An excess of fluid produced by the innermost of the fetal membranes (*amnion*) which forms the BAG OF WATERS that surrounds the fetus. *Acute hydramnios* is rare; it begins during mid-pregnancy and rapidly expands the uterus to enormous size. The condition terminates in spontaneous abortion or abortion induced to save the mother's life. *Chronic hydramnios* is a more common and less threatening form, does not often terminate in miscarriage, but frequently provokes premature labour
Hydrocele	Swelling of the scrotum from accumulation of fluid in the sac of the membrane that covers the testicles. It is painless but weight of the fluid causes a dragging sensation. Usually only one side is involved. The condition may be related to some injury but in most cases the cause is obscure and the testicles function normally. Chronic hydrocele, most frequent in middle-aged men, is relieved by withdrawal of fluid (TAPPING) but the swelling tends to recur. The sac can be removed surgically.
Hydrocephalus	Water on the brain; actually water *in* the brain – abnormal amounts of CEREBROSPINAL FLUID in brain cavities, exerting destructive pressure on brain substance.
Hydronephrosis	Swelling of the cavity of the kidney because of obstruction to outflow of urine, as from a stone, stricture, or tumour, in the kidney itself, in a ureter, or within the bladder.
Hydrophobia	See RABIES.
Hydrotherapy	Treatment by means of water.
Hymen	A membranous partition which partially blocks the external orifice of the virginal vagina.
Hyperbaric therapy	Treatment by inhalation of oxygen at greater than atmospheric pressure; an auxiliary to other appropriate treatment. The

patient, doctors, and nurses occupy a large chamber in which the atmospheric pressure is increased to about three times the sea level pressure. The patient breathes pure oxygen to increase the amount delivered to body cells. The technique has been employed experimentally in treatment of carbon monoxide poisoning, tetanus, and infections caused by bacteria which do not thrive in the presence of oxygen.

Excessive hydrochloric acid in gastric juice.	**Hyperchlorhydria**
Excessive amount of CHOLESTEROL in the blood.	**Hypercholesterol-aemia**
Vomiting of pregnancy, more severe than simple MORNING SICKNESS which clears up by itself; may require hospital treatment.	**Hyperemesis gravidarum**
Excessive sweating.	**Hyperhidrosis**
A condition of abnormally low blood sugar resulting from an excess of insulin or deficiency of sugar; similar to insulin shock.	**Hyperinsulism**
Longsightedness.	**Hypermetropia**
A malignant tumour of the kidney which occurs in persons over 40 years of age.	**Hypernephroma**
Overgrowth of an organ or tissue from an increase in the number of its cells which are, however, in normal arrangement.	**Hyperplasia**
Abnormally high arterial blood pressure.	**Hypertension**
A form of heart disease associated with high blood pressure which forces the heart to work harder to pump blood against resistance.	**Hypertensive heart disease**
Overactivity of the thyroid gland.	**Hyperthyroidism** (*thyrotoxicosis, toxic goitre*)
Increase in size of an organ, without an increase in the number	**Hypertrophy**

of cells. It is usually a response to increased activity or functional demands; voluntary, as when a much exercised muscle increases in size, or involuntary, as when the body enlarges one kidney to compensate for a deficiency of the other.

Hypnosis	Hypnosis is not a curative treatment, but at times can be helpful. Medical hypnosis first of all requires that the practitioner be trained as a doctor. The hypnotic trance itself is harmless but it can be misused by the medically untrained; a headache which can be temporarily hypnotized away may result from a brain tumour. The major medical uses of hypnosis are for relief of pain and anxiety; for example, in childbirth, dentistry, psychological preparation for anaesthesia and surgery. Hypnosis may reduce the amount of an anaesthetic that is needed, and is especially useful when anaesthetics and sedatives are for some reason undesirable. Unreasonably high hopes for medical hypnotic miracles are not justified.
Hypnotic	Inducing sleep; a sleeping pill.
Hypodermic	Under the skin; commonly refers to hypodermic injection, or the needle which effects it.
Hypoglycaemia	Deficiency of sugar in the blood. *Hypoglycaemic shock* due to an overdose of insulin is the same as *insulin shock*.
Hypo-ovarianism	Inadequate functioning of the ovaries.
Hypophysis	The pituitary gland.
Hypospadias	A congenital malformation in which the urethra, the urinary outlet, fails to fuse completely, but takes the form of an open troughlike channel on the underside of the penis. A similar malformation in the female permits urine to escape into the vagina.
Hypotension	Low blood pressure; sometimes significant, but usually harmless, not warranting treatment or concern, and indeed a factor in longevity.

A part of the brain concerned with primitive functions such as appetite, procreation, sleep, body temperature; closely associated with the pituitary gland.

Hypothalamus

Deficiency of thyroid hormone, leading to a slowing down of mental and physical processes. If the deficiency occurs in an infant before birth, it is known as *cretinism*; if it occurs in an adult, it is known as *myxoedema*.

Hypothyroidism

Surgical removal of the uterus, either through an abdominal incision or through the vagina, which leaves no abdominal scar.

Hysterectomy

I

Those unintentionally induced by words or actions of a doctor. A patient may misconstrue a doctor's remark or ominous look and be convinced that he has a grave disease which does not exist or is not nearly so grave as he fears. Iatrogenic heart disease is not uncommon; a doctor's casual mention of a murmur or premature beat may send a nervous patient into iatrogenic invalidism, although he would be much better off if he remained active. Some iatrogenic disease is unavoidable, the side effect of drugs which are necessary for the patient's welfare.	**Iatrogenic diseases**
Dry, fishlike scaliness of the skin, a congenital abnormality. There are two forms of ichthyosis, both of which are hereditary. The commoner form is transmitted as a dominant trait; the other is determined by a sex-linked recessive gene. The latter type affects males only but is transmitted by apparently normal females. It is not a danger to life or limb.	**Ichthyosis** (*fish skin disease*)
Same as JAUNDICE.	**Icterus**
Twins, always of the same sex and having the same heredity, developing from a single fertilized egg.	**Identical twins**
Originating spontaneously from unknown causes, not the result of any other disease; it is peculiar to the individual.	**Idiopathic**
Peculiar personal capacity to react differently from most people to drugs, foods, or treatment.	**Idiosyncrasy**
Inflammation of the ILEUM.	**Ileitis**
The lower portion of the small intestine, a tube several feet long in which major processes of digestion and assimilation take place. It is continuous with the *jejunum*, a section of the small intestine which lies above it, and joins the colon at the *caecum*, a pouch to which the appendix is attached. The *ileocaecal valve* at this junction controls the admission of its contents into the colon.	**Ileum**
The broad upper part of the pelvis.	**Ilium**

Immediate dentures	Artificial dentures worn immediately after extraction of the front teeth, the other teeth having been removed previously. While the gums are healing, the denture is prepared and is worn as soon as the front teeth are removed. This saves the patient the embarrassment of being conspicuously toothless for a while, and helps to prevent the gums from shrinking.
Immunity	Complex body mechanisms which create immunities to disease germs and foreign substances are not well understood, but research in this are has produced exciting knowledge which may ultimately be relevant to cancer, arthritis, and other diseases which many authorities think may be related to the inability of immunity mechanisms to cast out abnormal cells and substances. The role of the thymus in producing protective ANTIBODIES has only recently been clarified (see THYMUS GLAND). Immunity is partly humoral (that is, chemical) and partly cellular. There are two kinds of humoral immunity. *Passive immunity* is the kind borrowed from someone else, when a doctor injects GAMMA GLOBULIN or some other substance containing preformed antibodies made by another person or animal, or when a mother's antibodies are transferred to her unborn child. *Active immunity* is the kind produced by vaccination or exposure to disease germs; the body is stimulated to produce its own antibodies, continues to do so for a long time, and steps up antibody production when renewed by a booster dose or another contact with the same germs.
Immunization	Procedures by which immunities to diseases are produced in a person; especially, by vaccines and toxoids. See IMMUNITY, *active* and *passive*.
Immunoglobulins	Substances in the blood and in other body fluids which build immunities to various diseases; loosely synonymous with ANTIBODIES.
Impacted	Firmly lodged, wedged in place; as, an impacted wisdom tooth, embedded in the jawbone.
Imperforate hymen	Complete closure of the membrane at the opening of the vagina.

Incapacity of the male to have a penile erection and perform the sexual act. Impotence is an impediment of delivery rather than of production of SPERMATOZOA; it is not the same as infertility, which may affect perfectly potent males. Anatomical defects, injuries, or disorders of the nervous or endocrine systems, and systemic diseases may cause impotence, and the possibility should first be investigated. But the majority of cases have a psychological basis; the affected male may be impotent with one sexual partner but not with another; emotional factors are varied and complex, and counselling or psychiatric help may be required.

Impotence

The four cutting teeth at the front of the upper and lower-jaws.

Incisors

Inability to retain urine or faeces.

Incontinence

The time between infection with disease organisms and the first appearance of symptoms. The period varies for different diseases, as short as a day or two for influenza and as long as 100 days for serum hepatitis.

Incubation period

A tiny anvil-shaped bone, the middle bone in the chain of *ossicles* of the middle ear which conduct sounds to the inner ear.

Incus

A general lay term for abdominal distress with such symptoms as heartburn, distension, gas, cramps, and fullness.

Indigestion

Artificial stimulation of labour before it starts naturally; accomplished by rupturing the BAG OF WATERS, use of drugs such as *oxytocin*, or mechanical means.

Induction of labour

An eruptive skin disorder of infancy, frequently due to food sensitivities.

Infantile eczema

Newborn infants do not sleep most of the time. They sleep about 16 hours out of 24, and can sleep only about four hours at a stretch. One study of newborn infants showed only a gradual decrease in amount of sleep per day over a 16-week

Infant sleep patterns

period. By the time they were four months of age they slept about 14½ hours a day, while increasing the length of a single sleep period to a little more than eight hours. Waking periods of newborn infants are more frequent from 5 p.m. to 3 a.m. than during the day. Long intervals between feedings may account for night-time wakefulness. At two to three weeks of age, CIRCADIAN RHYTHMS (24-hour cycles) of sleep and wakefulness begin to develop. At three years of age a child has generally consolidated his sleep time and sleeps about ten hours a night. Difficulties in sleeping may be aggravated about the fifth year when daytime naps are given up. There is no arbitrary time for giving up afternoon naps, but generally they should be tapered off when a nap delays the onset of sleep in the evening and keeps the child awake after going to bed.

Infarct	An area of dead tissue resulting from complete blockage of its blood supply. This frequently occurs in *coronary thrombosis* when a clot in a coronary artery stops the supply of blood to a portion of the heart muscle, producing *myocardial infarction.*
Infectious jaundice	See LEPTOSPIROSIS.
Infectious mononucleosis	An infection thought to be caused by the Epstein-Barr (EB) virus. It generally lasts about two weeks; patients with the most acute symptoms require on the average only four days of bed rest, the majority require no bed rest, but there may be relapses.
Inflammation	Inflammation is a defensive reaction to all sorts of tissue injury. The names of inflammatory processes are designated by the suffix '-itis," preceded by the name of the affected tissue – for example, *appendicitis, arthritis*. The four characteristics of inflammation are reddening, swelling, pain, and heat. Reddening results from increased blood supply to the affected parts; white blood cells whose job it is to trap and destroy germs are also increased. Concentration of fluids causes swelling. Increase of blood supply and local metabolism produces heat. Pain is a warning not to abuse the part and to get something done about it. A doctor is needed if inflammation

is at all serious, to find out what is wrong and what to do about it.

An acute highly infectious viral disease tending to occur in epidemics.	**Influenza** (*grippe, flu*)
Introduction of fluid into a vein.	**Infusion**
Curled, corkscrew-like hairs that burrow into the skin, particularly affecting the bearded area. Shaving may cut such hairs more or less longitudinally, leaving a sharp point which turns in upon its owner. The ingrown hair may cause inflammation of the follicle, and the usual treatment is to pull it out with antiseptic precautions	**Ingrown hairs**
Of or relating to the GROIN. A frequent site of hernia.	**Inguinal**
Introduction of a disease agent into the body to produce a mild form of the disease, giving immunity; for example, cowpox vaccination for smallpox.	**Inoculation**
Introduction of semen into the vagina, by natural means or by artifical insemination.	**Insemination**
In a normal place.	**In situ**
Inhaling, breathing in.	**Inspiration**
Thickened, from absorption or evaporation of fluid.	**Inspissated**
Blowing gas or powder into a body cavity, as the lungs or vagina.	**Insufflation**
A hormone produced by the islet cells of the pancreas, essential for metabolism. Insulin in treatment of *diabetes* must be given by injection, since it is a protein molecule broken down by digestion. Pharmaceutical companies prepare insulin in a number of different forms from animal sources. The structure of insulin was worked out by Frederick Sanger, a British biochemist. Insulin is a rather small protein molecule com-	**Insulin**

posed of 51 amino acids in two chains held together by sulphur links. Human and animal insulins have the same properties but differ in a sequence of three amino acids in one of the chains.

Intention tremor

Involuntary movements caused or intensified by voluntary movement.

Intercostal

Between the ribs.

Interferon

Infection caused by one virus may prevent concurrent infection by another virus. This phenomenon is called viral interference. An apparent mechanism which gives this protection has recently come under study. It is now known that body cells invaded by a virus produce a substance called *interferon* which diffuses out of the cells and into neighbouring cells. The cells then become resistant to infection by viruses. Interferon is a complex protein. Its production by the body is a generalized phenomenon occurring when cells are exposed to viruses. Its unique properties suggest that it might be developed into an agent for treatment of viral diseases, but great practical difficulties stand in the way. Interferon is too complex for synthetic manufacture and difficulties of producing large amounts of the pure substance are formidable. Even if interferon becomes available, its medical uses would be limited. Interferon must be absorbed into cells to block the multiplication of viruses, and means must be found to get interferon into cells in time to produce a curative or beneficial response.

Intermenstrual pain

A usually brief attack of moderate to severe pain which some women experience about midway between menstrual periods, coincidental with OVULATION, rupture of an egg-sac of the ovary and release of a mature ovum. Primary DYSMENORRHOEA never occurs in the absence of ovulation; intermenstrual pain of this nature is a rough guide to the time of ovulation and the fertile period. Discovery in 1940 that ovulation is essential for menstrual cramps, and that administration of oestrogen early in the cycle could eliminate the cramps, later led to the development of oral contraceptive pills. The right ovary lies near the appendix and midmenstrual pain in that region may be mistaken for a symptom of appendicitis. A doctor can distinguish between intermenstrual pain and appendicitis on the basis of laboratory tests and dates of the menstrual cycle.

Pain in the calf muscles and limping on exercise, due to inadequate blood supply.

Intermittent claudication

See HERMAPHRODITE.

Intersex

Redness, abrasion, and maceration of opposing skin surfaces that rub together. Common sites are the armpit, groin, anal region, and beneath the breasts. Moisture and warmth with friction of adjacent skin set the stage of chafing, which may be complicated by bacterial or fungus infection. Cleanliness, regular use of a dusting powder, and reduction in weight if obese are helpful preventives. Diabetes increases the susceptibility to intertrigo.

Intertrigo (*chafing*)

Cartilaginous cushions between vertebrae.

Intervertebral discs

Bacteria which normally inhabit the intestine, do no harm, and in fact are helpful. Varieties of intestinal bacteria vary somewhat with diet. Diseases or antibiotics or other circumstances sometimes incapacitate one or more floral species, permitting others to thrive disproportionately from lack of competition; this may cause disturbing symptoms. A few kinds of bacteria may get through the stomach, but most kinds do not survive the antiseptic acid gastric juices. The floral population flourishes increasingly from the stomach downwards. Some intestinal bacteria synthesize all the vitamin K we need, some synthesize other B vitamins, but not all these products are well absorbed.

Intestinal flora

Digestive juices secreted by the intestinal walls, in contrast to gastric juices secreted by the stomach, and pancreatic juices secreted by the pancreas. Intestinal juices contain enzymes which complete the final stages in digestion of protein, fat, and carbohydrate.

Intestinal juices

Intestine	The digestive tube from the outlet of the stomach to the outlet of the rectum. Although it is a continuous structure, each of the different sections has a different function. See DUODENUM, JEJUNUM, ILEUM, CAECUM, COLON, RECTUM.
Intima	The inner lining of an artery; the innermost of its three coats or layers.
Intracutaneous test	Introduction of allergens into the skin; a positive reaction indicating sensitivity to a test substance will manifest itself in a few minutes in the form of an itching skin eruption.
Intradermal	Into or within the skin.
Intramuscular	Into or within a muscle. Some drugs are injected into muscles, usually the buttocks.
Intrauterine contraceptive devices (IUD, IUCD)	Flexible devices of stainless steel, silk-worm gut, or plastic, inserted by a doctor into the uterus and retained there indefinitely for prevention of conception. Various devices are shaped like a bow, spiral, ring, or loop.
Intravenous (*I.V.*)	Into or within a vein; as, *intravenous feeding*.
Intrinsic factor	A substance produced by the stomach for the transport of vitamin B_{12}, across membranes into the blood. The fundamental defect in *pernicious anaemia* is absence or deficiency of intrinsic factor so that vitamin B_{12}, necessary for normal development of red blood cells, cannot be absorbed from foods.
Intubation	Introduction of a tube into a hollow organ such as the larynx,
Intussusception	Sliding of a part of the intestine into its hollow interior; telescoping, like the pushed-in finger of a glove.
In vitro	Literally, in glass; of or relating to studies done in test tubes or by laboratory methods, outside the living body. *In vivo* studies are done with living persons or organisms.

Ionizing Radiation

The effect of radiation (X-rays, radium, radioisotopes, and so on) is to drive electrons out of atoms or molecules, forming chemical units called *ions*. Such alteration of the electron patterns of components of living cells, changing their functional capacities, is the basis for the therapeutic use of X-rays.

Iridectomy

Excision of a piece of the iris to open drainage channels for relief of *glaucoma*.

Iris

The circular, pigmented structure of the eye, perforated by the pupil. The iris controls the amount of light entering the eye and gives the eyes their colour. *Iritis* is an inflammation of the iris.

Iron

The essential mineral of HAEMOGLOBIN. The body preserves its iron stores, and constantly reuses iron salvaged from broken-down red blood cells. The small amount lost each day is replaced from the diet, but if reserves are severely depleted, food alone will not restore them. Infants and children particularly need good sources of iron; milk, which may constitute a large proportion of their diet, is relatively low in iron and paediatrician's advice about addition of solid foods or possible supplements should be followed. Pregnancy increases a woman's requirements for iron; supplements are usually given. Chronic blood loss, dietary deficiencies, or disorders of absorption may result in iron-deficiency anaemia. It is easy for a doctor to determine if iron-deficiency anaemia exists in a patient. Unless it does, iron will do nothing to correct fatigue or a possibly serious underlying disease of which fatigue is a symptom. In men, iron-deficiency anaemia leads the doctor to look for some cause of chronic blood loss, such as bleeding ulcer or haemorrhoids. Women of childbearing age are more susceptible to iron-deficiency anaemia because of monthly blood losses, but the loss normally is very small in terms of iron. *Good food sources of iron* Whole grain and enriched cereals   Dried beans and peas   Greens   Eggs   Apricots   Meat and poultry   Liver and kidney   Prunes and raisins   Molasses   Dried figs and peaches   Bouillon cubes   Brewer's yeast   Wheat germ   Nuts

Iron lung	Popular name for a machine which expands and contracts the chest, so that a person with paralysed respiratory muscles can breathe; a respirator.
Iron poisoning	Common iron pills or tablets, prescribed for iron-deficiency anaemia and commonly for pregnant women, are dangerous and even deadly to small children who get hold of a bottle and swallow the pills which sometimes look like sweets. Children have died from swallowing such tablets, usually five-grain tablets of ferrous sulphate. Symptoms of poisoning develop in an hour or so, with signs of shock, coma, vomiting, diarrhoea. Iron poisoning is an acute emergency requiring immediate medical treatment. So keep all medicines locked away from children.
Irradiation, *medical*	Treatment or diagnosis of disease with X-rays, RADIOISOTOPES, or other sources of IONIZING RADIATION. The body normally contains a certain amount of radioactive potassium and is subject to radiation from rocks and other unavoidable background sources.
Irreducible	Incapable of being put back into the normal position; said of a hernia.
Irregation	Washing out of a cavity.
Irritable bowel syndrome	Overreaction of the colon to emotions or other stimuli, without discoverable organic cause. Symptoms include pain in the lower abdomen, distension, and abdominal aching.
Ischaemia	Local deficiency of blood supply, due to spasm or obstruction of an artery. A frequent concomitant of *coronary artery disease*.
Ischium	One of the bones of the pelvis. The bone we sit on.
Islet cells	The cells of the pancreas which produce INSULIN. Also called *islets of Langerhans*.
Isometric exercise	A form of exercise in which a muscle group exerts utmost force

without moving a part. No special equipment is needed. Muscles of the abdomen or other parts of the body can be held at maximum tension while sitting or standing; arms can push against the sides of a doorway while standing in the opening; the palms of the hands can strain upward under the kneehold space of a desk while one sits in front of it. Isometric exercise builds strength up to a plateau. After the plateau is reached, increasing frequency of exercise does not increase strength further. Mild effort is useless. Strength increases only if maximum effort is maintained for a least six seconds.

Intravenous.   I.V.

A *focal* epileptic seizure, so called because the spasm or convulsion originates in a local part of the brain and its effects are limited to one part of the body; for example, a twitching arm or leg.	**Jacksonian seizure**
A virus-caused infection, occurring in eastern Asia, transmitted by the bites of mosquitoes.	**Japanese encephalitis**
Yellow discoloration of the skin and tissues by bile pigments in the blood. The skin may itch. The urine is dark yellow or brown. The whites of the eyes have a yellowish tinge; in skin discolorations which might be mistaken for jaundice, the whites of the eyes remain clear. The symptom indicates that something has happened to cause bile pigments to mount up in the blood. The underlying abnormality may be in the liver, in the bile passages outside the liver, or in the blood itself. *Haemolytic jaundice* is due to increased destruction of red blood cells; the stools are dark. A harmless form of haemolytic jaundice occurs in newborn babies and lasts for three or four days; the baby has an excess of red cells which are destroyed during the first few days after birth. *Toxic* or *infective jaundice* reflects injury to liver cells by some agent which interferes with their ability to eliminate bile pigment. *Obstructive jaundice* results when bile ducts are blocked by disease, inflammation, gallstones, infection, or tumours. In this type of jaundice the discoloration of skin and mucous membranes is intense, the stools clay-coloured, and the urine deeply coloured. Underlying causes of jaundice are numerous. Various laboratory tests help to detect what is wrong.	**Jaundice**
A peptic ulcer occurring near the opening between the stomach and jejunum, after a surgical operation to establish a direct connection between the organs (*gastrojejunostomy*).	**Jejunal ulcer**
A portion of the small intestine, several feet long, continuous from the DUODENUM to the ILEUM. Absorption of food is practically limited to the small intestine. Digestion is accelerated in the jejunum which is the recipient of gruel-like materials from the stomach after thorough mixing with bile and pancreatic juices in the duodenum.	**Jejunum**

Jellyfish stings
See PORTUGUESE MAN-OF-WAR.

Jet injection
A technique for vaccinating without a needle. A volume of liquid is suddenly compressed and forced through a very fine orifice at such speed that it penetrates the skin painlessly and delivers a cone-shaped spray of material into the tissues under the skin. Various types of jet injectors have been developed; some have reservoirs holding enough material for several hundred doses. The devices have been used principally for mass vaccination of large numbers of people.

Jiggers
Sand fleas; pregnant females of the species bore into the skin, causing intense itching and inflammation.

Joint mice
Small loose fragments of bone that have become separated within a joint, often the knee.

Joule
The unit of energy. Has largely replaced the Calorie in dietetics.

Jugular veins
Veins of the side of the neck which drain blood from the head and neck towards the heart. The internal jugular veins are deep-lying; the external ones are near the surface.

K

A blood test for syphilis.	**Kahn test**
An infection transmitted by the bites of sandflies, occurring in Mediterranean, tropical, and oriental regions. It is characterised by fever, anaemia, enlarged spleen, emaciation, and has a high fatality rate if left untreated, but responds well to medical treatment.	**Kala-azar**
See XERODERMA PIGMENTOSUM.	**Kaposi's disease**
Irregular ridges, nodules, and cordlike bands of skin like raised scars, at first rubbery and later very dense and hard. They tend to occur on the site of previous scars. The cause of such excessive growth is not known. Keloids can be removed by surgery or shrunk by radiation, but have a tendency to recur.	**Keloids**
The hard, horny protein which is the chief structural material of the outermost layer of the skin, of hair and nails, and in animals lower than man, of claws, horns, hooves, and feathers.	**Keratin**
Inflammation of the cornea.	**Keratitis**
Acute inflammation of the cornea and conjuctiva, tending to occur in epidemics, caused by a specific virus.	**Keratoconjunctivitis**
Cone-shaped projection of the cornea; vision impaired by the bending of light waves in distorted ways. Good vision may be restored by contact lenses.	**Keratoconus**
Surgical procedures on the cornea, such as CORNEAL TRANSPLANT.	**Keratoplasty**
Overgrowth of the horny layer of the skin; for example, a wart or callus.	**Keratosis**
Fungus infection of the beard or scalp, producing pustules.	**Kerion**
A severe form of JAUNDICE characterized by deposits of bile	**Kernicterus**

pigments in parts of the brain and degeneration of nerve cells, occurring in infants with ERYTHROBLASTOSIS.

Ketosis

A condition produced when more fat is eaten than can be burned completely by the body. The unburned fats produce acid chemical substances called *ketone bodies*. An excess of ketones produces a form of ACIDOSIS to which some diabetics are especially susceptible; acetone derived from incomplete combustion of fats can produce a characteristic odour to the breath of diabetics with *ketoacidosis*.

Kidneys

Paired organs in the small of the back behind the abdominal cavity. The kidneys regulate the volumes and composition of the body fluids, filter out impurities, keep ELECTROLYTES and blood composition in balance, and secrete substances which modify blood pressure. The kidneys are subject to infections, stone formation, tumours, malformations, circulatory and other diseases.

Kimmelsteil-Wilson disease (*diabetic nephropathy*)

A specific form of kidney disease (scerosis of the GLOMERULI) associated with diabetes of long duration.

Kinaesthesia

The sense by which we perceive weight, position, movement, resistance, and rapidly integrate countless muscle-registered stimuli – from a grasped steering wheel, tennis racket, bicycle handlebars, or from muscles that tell us an arm is outstretched or bent without our looking at it.

Kinins

Miniature proteins associated with rheumatism and allergic reactions.

Kiss ulcer

One that appears to result from parts that press upon or are in contact with each other.

Klebsiella pneumonia

A type of pneumonia caused by a type of bacteria other than the common pneumococci. It tends to produce chronic lung abscesses.

Klinefelter's syndrome

Undeveloped testes and female characteristics such as breast enlargement in males, due to an abnormality of the sex-determining pair of CHROMOSOMES. A normal female has two X chromosomes (XX), a normal male, an X and a Y (XY). A person with Klinefelter's syndrome has an extra and harmful X chromosome (XXY).

A blood test for syphilis.	**Kline test**

The patellar reflex; sudden jerking forward of the lower leg when tapped below the kneecap. A test of the integrity of nerves.	**Kneejerk**

Inward bending of the knees at the joint; in young children it usually corrects itself spontaneously.	**Knock-knees** *(genu valgum)*

Small bluish-white spots on mucous membranes of the cheeks, present shortly before the rash of MEASLES appears.	**Koplik's spots**

This servere mental disturbance usually, but not always, follows a bout of DELIRIUM TREMENS which blends into it. The outstanding manifestation is loss of memory for recent events, and falsifications of memory, such as remembering things that never happened. The psychosis is associated with chronic alcoholism and chronic malnutrition; treatment is much the same as for delirium tremens. Some patients recover their memories after weeks or months, but others never do.	**Korsakoff's psychosis**

Progressive drying and shrivelling of the skin, due to atrophy of glands, often accompanied by severe itching; especially, kraurosis of the vulva in elderly women.	**Kraurosis**

A PROTEIN deficiency disease occurring most often in children in tropical countries who are raised on cereal diets after weaning. Affected children have pot bellies, apathy, muscular wasting, oedema, and fail to grow. It is an extreme form of disease which may occur in lesser degree in persons whose diets are very low in protein. The basic deficiency is lack of AMINO ACIDS for synthesis of proteins.	**Kwashiorkor**

Humpback curvature of the spine. A mild form is round shoulders. Kyphosis may result from poor posture or from	**Kyphosis**

L

Lips or liplike organs. *Labia majora*, folds of skin on either side of the entrance of the vulva; *labia minora*, folds of tissue covered with mucous membrane within the labia majora.	**Labia**
Childbirth. There are three stages: dilation of the cervix; expulsion of the child; expulsion of the placenta.	**Labour**
Intricate passageways, intercommunicating canals; especially, structures of the inner ear.	**Labyrinth**
A wound caused by tearing of tissue; for example, laceration of the perineum in childbirth.	**Laceration**
Of or relating to tears, produced by the *lacrinmal gland* in the upper outer region of the orbit.	**Lacrimal**
Secretion of milk. Interacting hormones initiate and sustain this complicated process. The milk-duct system of the breast enlarges during pregnancy under the influence of *oestrogen*, an ovarian hormone. Milk-secreting lobules also proliferate under the influence of a different hormone, *progesterone*. During labour, OXYTOCIN, another hormone, takes effect. Shortly after the baby is born the breasts secrete COLOSTRUM, which is not true milk but a secretion containing protective antibodies of the mother. True milk appears when *prolactin*, a pituitary gland hormone, acts upon breasts already prepared by oestrogen and progesterone. Lactation can be suppressed by giving suitable hormones.	**Lactation**
The sugar of milk.	**Lactose**
A person who lives on a diet of vegetables, cereals, fruits, and dairy products.	**Lactovegetarian**
The most common form of cirrhosis of the liver; portal cirrhosis.	**Laennec's cirrhosis**
Surgical opening of the wall of the spinal canal to expose underlying structures.	**Laminectomy**

Lancet	A short, pointed, double-edged surgical knife, used for *lancing* – that is, cutting open.
Lancinating	A description of sharply cutting, shooting pain.
Lanugo	Fine downy hair on the body of the fetus and on the adult body, except the palms and soles.
Laparotomy	Opening of the abdomen by an incision; a variety of surgical procedures may be used subsequent to the opening.
Larva migrans	See CREEPING ERUPTION.
Laryngectomy	Surgical removal of all or part of the voice box, usually because of cancer. There is a high rate of cure if the cancer is discovered early. The patient is left without vocal cords, but with persistence and encouragement can learn to speak again by swallowing and belching air and manipulating it with muscles of the tongue and mouth.
Laryngitis	Inflammation of the LARYNX (voice box). Acute laryngitis is often associated with a common cold, infection, or overuse of the voice. The throat is dry, swallowing may be affected, it is not possible to speak above a hoarse whisper, if at all. Absolute rest of the voice is an essential part of treatment.
Laryngoscope	A hollow metal tube with a light, inserted into the throat for examining the LARYNX.
Laryngotracheo-bronchitis	An acute, serious condition of children, rapid in onset, requiring immediate medical care. The outstanding symptom is extreme difficulty in breathing, due to thick mucus and fluid which can plug the breathing passages.
Larynx	The vocal apparatus, located between the base of the tongue and the windpipe. It includes the vocal cords and muscles which modify the vibrations of air passing through them, to produce controlled sounds.

L

Laser

A device which gets its name from the initial letters of Light Amplification by Stimulated Emission of Radiation. Essentially, a laser multiples the energy of a light source, such as the flash of a photographic bulb, into a very powerful emission of parallel light waves of the same wavelength, all in step. The original laser employed a ruby crystal about the size of a cigarette, impregnated with chromium atoms, with a reflective mirror at one end and a semitransparent mirror at the other. Setting off a high-powered flash bulb excites atoms in the crystal to higher energy levels; they drop to normal levels and in doing so excite other atoms, trapped between mirrored ends of the tube, rebounding, intensifying, until an extremely intense burst of coherent (nondiffuse) light is emitted from the semitransparent end of the tube. For a very brief time, hundredths of thousands of a second, a laser beam is more brilliant than the sun and its parallel rays can be focused on a spot no wider than a millionth of a millimetre. Medical uses of a laser are still experimental and many problems remain to be solved. Laser beams have successfully destroyed pigmented skin cancers in human patients, have been used to remove portwine stains and tattoos, and have been employed to secure *detached retinas* into position.

Laurence-Moon-Biedl syndrome

A rare genetic disorder of the pituitary gland, producing obesity, mental retardation, degeneration of the retina, webbed fingers or toes and underdevelopment of the genitals.

Lavage

Washing out of a hollow organ such as the stomach or a sinus.

Lead poisoning

Intoxication from absorption of lead or its salts into the body; *Plumbism*. Mild lead poisoning may produce no apparent symptoms but the metal can accumulate in the body over a period of time and produce chronic poisoning. Some of the signs of lead poisoning are abdominal pain, constipation, muscle weakness, pallor, drowsiness, mental confusion, and a blue line on the gums. Lead poisoning occasionally occurs in young children who chew objects containing paints with a lead base. Insidious lead poisoning is not rare in children who live in old, poorly maintained houses with flaking paint and plaster. Fortunately, lead paint is little used now. Infants explore the world by putting all sorts of things into their mouths. About the time when they begin to walk and have a few teeth, they may develop an abnormal appetite for non-food substances (see PICA). It is a dangerous habit which should be corrected by teaching the child as early as possible what should and should not go into his mouth.

L E cell

A white blood cell which has undergone changes characteristic of *lupus erythematosus* and related diseases.

Left-handedness

When a left-handed child appears in a right-handed family there may be some worry. The left-handed may suffer unjustly in a right-handed world. Perhaps it is such considerations that lead some parents to force a naturally left-handed child to favour his right hand. The consensus of medical opinion is that if a child wants to use his left hand, let him. Some things we learn to do with either the right or left hand because it is more convenient. A left-handed person shakes hands with his right hand because that is the way the world shakes hands. A right-handed person holds a telephone receiver with his left hand and uses his left ear to leave his right hand free for writing. We are left- or right-eyed as well as handed; it is easy to determine one's dominant eye. Teachers and parents never make any effort to change eye dominance. If handedness is to some extent hereditary, the mode of transmission has not been elucidated.

Leishmaniasis

A parasitic disease transmitted by sandflies; it has several forms.

Leprosy
(*Hansen's disease*)

A chronic disease which inflicts deformities and multilations, caused by bacteria closely related to those that cause tuberculosis. About twelve million people suffer from leprosy today. Most of them live in tropical or subtropical countries. The disease affects the skin and nerves of all patients, but is usually classified according to which tissue is predominantly involved. Patients with nerve leprosy develop discoloured skin areas, devoid of feeling because nerves are deadened. Ultimately, fingers, toes, or other parts may shrivel. Patients with skin leprosy develop thick swellings which grossly distort the features. Drugs known as sulphones seem to prolong the lives of some patients but others appear to get worse after chemotherapy is begun. Close skin contact with a patient who has leprosy seems a likely route of entry of organisms into the body. Leprosy is generally thought not to be very catching. Husbands and wives of patients with leprosy may remain apparently uninfected after living many years together. Some investigators feel that leprosy is a highly contagious disease but only to a few people who are highly susceptible.

An infectious disease caused by certain spirochaetes (*leptospira*). The germs are spread in the urine of infected animals – rats, mice, dogs, cows, pigs – and most people who acquire the infection have had contact with animals or with water or moist soil to which animals have access. Several local outbreaks have been traced to swimming or wading in ponds or slow-moving streams in rural areas where waste disposal is not properly screened. The germs enter the body through mucous membranes or minute breaks in the skin. Typically, the infection produces sudden fever, chills, headache, and muscle pains. In some cases there may be few if any symptoms; in others, jaundice may develop. Usually leptospirosis is a brief self-limited illness, but *Weil's disease* is a severe form in which jaundice, kidney failure, haemorrhage, anaemia, and heart damage may beome threatening complications. Leptospirosis responds well to antibiotics.	**Leptospirosis** (*infectious jaundice;* *spirochaetal jaundice*)
Alteration of tissue or function due to injury or disease. A pimple, fracture, abscess, scratch, wart, or ingrowing toenail may be called a lesion.	**Lesion**
White blood cells.	**Leucocytes**
Abnormal increase in numbers of white blood cells. The cell count normally increases slightly after eating and in pregnancy, but the word implies an abnormal increase, often associated with bodily defences against infection and inflammation. For instance, a high count may help to confirm a diagnosis of appendicitis. Disorders of the blood-forming organs may also induce leucocytosis	**Leucocytosis**

Leucopenia

Diminished number of white blood cells. The condition may result from allergies, drug reactions, irradiation, certain kinds of infections, or anaemias.

Leucorrhoea

Whitish discharge from the vagina. Increased flow of mucus about midway between menstrual periods often accompanies OVULATION. The discharge is sometimes called the whites. It may also result from yeast or protozoal infection. See TRICHOMONIASIS and CANDIDIASIS.

Leukaemia

Malignant disease of the blood-forming organs. The characteristic abnormality is gross overproduction of white blood cells. There are several acute and chronic forms of leukaemia, so diverse that the word does not refer to a single specific disease but to a variety of leukaemia states.

Leukoderma

SEE VITILIGO

Leukoplakia

Whitish leathery patches on mucous membranes of the mouth or vulva. No specific cause is known, but continued irritation is considered to be a factor. Patients with oral leukoplakia are forbidden to smoke and the white patches may regress if this and other irritations are removed. Leukoplakia by no means progresses inevitably to cancer, but it is considered to be a precancerous lesion and requires medical care and supervision.

Leydig cells

Interstitial cells of the testes which produce testosterone, the male hormone (and small amounts of female hormone). The cells are separate structures from those that produce SPERMATOZOA. Thus, infertile males whose production of spermatozoa is impaired may produce adaquate amounts of male hormone and be normally potent.

LH

Luteinizing hormone of the pituitary gland. It causes a GRAAFIAN FOLLICLE which has released an egg to become a yellow body which produces progesterone, a hormone which helps to prepare the lining of the uterus for implantation of a fertilized egg.

L

Commonly means sexual desire.	**Libido**
Leathery thickening and hardening of the skin, usually the result of long-continued irritation from scratching and rubbing.	**Lichenification**
An itching eruption of unknown cause; dull purplish-red spots appear on thin-skinned areas of the body.	**Lichen planus**
A band of tough, flexible fibrous tissue which connects bones or supports organs.	**Ligament**
To tie up; for example, a bleeding blood vessel. In surgery, a ligature is a thread of silk, catgut, wire, or other material used for tying vessels.	**Ligate**
The time around the middle of the last month of pregnancy when the baby's head settles more deeply into the pelvis preparatory to birth. This slightly decreases the mother's feeling of abdominal distension.	**Lightening**
A border; the edge of the cornea where it joins the white of the eye.	**Limbus**
A broad term for fats and fatlike substances. Lipids contain one or more fatty acids. Lipids include fats, cholesterol, phospholipids, and similar substances which do not mix readily with water.	**Lipids**
See ASPIRATION PNEUMONIA.	**Lipoid pneumonia**
A tumour composed of fat tissue, occuring chiefly on the trunk, back of the neck, forearms, or armpits. Lipomas must be distinguished from other tumours. Lipomas usually stop growing after they reach a certain size and remain at that size indefinitely. True lipomas are painless, harmless, never become malignant, and are best left untreated unless they are so large and cosmetically objectionable as to justify surgical removal.	**Lipoma**

Lithiasis	Stone formation (gallstones, kidney stones); the condition of having stones.
Lithotomy	Cutting into the bladder to remove a stone. Structures are close to the surface, and because of this accessibility the operation has an ancient history. Mortality was high in the centuries before antiseptic surgery, but some patients did recover.
Little's disease	Cerebral palsy of children, affecting both sides of the body.
Liver fluke	A disease acquired by ingesting food or water contaminated with cysts of sheep liver flukes, a species of flatworm.
Lobotomy	Cutting into a lobe of an organ, especially a lobe of the brain.
Lochia	The discharge from the vagina which continues for a week or two after childbirth. It is a normal aftermath of childbirth and ceases when the uterus returns to its pre-pregnancy state.
Locked knee	A painfully swollen knee joint which cannot be extended fully, due to a torn CARTILAGE. Surgical removal of the injured cartilage is usually necessary.
Lockjaw	See TETANUS
Locomotor ataxia	See ATAXIA
Longsightedness (hypermetropia)	A condition in which light from near objects is focused behind rather than upon the retina, usually because the eyeball is too short. Close objects are blurred but distant ones are distinct. Longsighted persons may read and do close work with some success through ACCOMODATION, but this effort of ciliary muscles can give rise to complaints of eye strain, tired eyes, and distaste for tasks of close seeing. With increasing age, the lens of the eye loses flexibility and longsighted people tend to hold their newspapers at arm's length to read them. Glasses for reading, or a reading segment in bifocal glasses, can do much to give comfort.

L

Exaggeration of the normal forward curve of the spine at the small of the back. The general aspect is that of an abdomen thrust forward and shoulders thrust back. The characteristic posture of late pregnancy is a lordosis. Abnormalities of the hip joint sometimes cause lordosis.	**Lordosis**
Less than normal amounts of glucose (sugar) in circulating blood. Blood sugar naturally drops if there is a .long interval between meals. Mild transient symptoms of hunger, weakness, faintness, are perfectly normal and no surprise to anyone who omits food long enough to deplete his reserves; a meal restores the balance. *Chronic* hypoglycaemia may be associated with various endocrine and other disorders. Insulin, which reduces abnormally high blood sugar levels, is only one agent in nature's complicated balancing scheme. Another hormone, *glucagon*, also produced by the pancreas, but by different cells from those which produce insulin, stimulates the liver to convert GLYCOGEN to blood sugar and raise low blood sugar levels.	**Low blood sugar** (HYPOGLYCAEMIA)
Lysergic acid diethylamide.	**LSD**
Syphilis.	**Lues**
A general term for pain in the lumbar region. Lumbago is not a specific disease but a sympton to be investigated.	**Lumbago**
Withdrawal of CEREBROSPINAL FLUID through a hollow needle inserted between lumbar vertebrae of the small of the back. Withdrawal may be done for purposes of diagnosis, to relieve pressure, or the puncture may be made to introduce medication, such as an anaesthetic.	**Lumbar puncture**
The open space inside a tubular structure such as an intestine or blood vessel.	**Lumen**
Dislocation.	**Luxation**
Inflammation of lymphatic vessels due to spread of an infection. Red lines mark the paths of inflamed vessels. There is a	**Lymphangitis**

danger of bacteria getting into the blood. Treatment is directed to overcoming the original infection.

Lymphoedema

Swelling of a part of the body, especially the legs or arms, from accumulation of fluids because of obstruction or inadequacy of the lymphatic drainage system. The condition may cause huge enlargement of a part (ELEPHANTIASIS) Lymphoedema of the arm sometimes occurs after breast removal surgery. Obstructive lymphoedema is secondary to other conditions such as tumours or FILARIASIS. A less frequent, sometimes congenital form results from primary defects in the functioning of lymphatic channels in the skin and its deep layers. This type of lymphoedema manifests itself as a grossly swollen leg in the teens or middle life. The unsightly swelling may be controlled to some degree by rest in bed, elevation of the limb to promote drainage, and wearing a firm rubber bandage over a stocking when up and about. However, this does not cure a chronic condition which tends to worsen with time, and surgery to remove the diseased tissue before extensive changes occur may be advisable.

Lymphogranuloma venereum

A disease produced by viruses transmitted by sexual contact.

Lymphosarcoma

A malignant tumour of lymphatic tissue. *Lymphogranulomatosis* is sometimes a synonym for HODGKIN'S DISEASE.

Lysozyme

A natural antibacterial substance contained in some bodily secretions, such as tears.

Softening and deterioration of tissue in constant confined contact with fluids.	**Maceration**
A small, round, yellowish spot near the centre of the retina; the area of colour perception and most distinct vision.	**Macula lutea**
A flat discoloured spot on the surface of the skin. The rash of measles is macular.	**Macule**
A chronic fungus infection of the foot, occuring in tropical regions. The swollen foot becomes filled with connecting cystlike areas from which fungus-containing pus drains. In time the disease destroys the tissues, and amputation may be necessary.	**Madura foot** (*mycetoma*)
The HYMEN.	**Maidenhead**
A descriptive term for several disorders resulting from defective absorption of foodstuffs in the small intestine. Certain diseases or surgical procedures may disturb previously normal assimilative processes, but the most common forms of the syndrome (variously called *coeliac disease, sprue, idiopathic steatorrhoea*) seem to involve hereditary defects in the absorptive surface of the small intestine, and dificient activity of intestinal enzymes. Large amounts of unabsorbed fat produce frequent, pale, loose stools (*steatorrhoea*), *Coeliac disease* in children is the same as *nontropical sprue* in adults. Symptoms in adults – diarrhoea, weakness, loss of weight, anaemia deceptively like pernicious anaemia – are insidious and require careful diagnosis. Young children with coeliac disease commonly have poor appetite, various signs of malnutrition, stunted growth, bulging abdomen, and frequent frothy stools containing excessive amounts of fat. Gluten, a wheat protein, has a toxic effect on the small bowel of many patients with malabsorption syndromes. Strict elimination of gluten from the diet often restores bowel function to normal and maintains it even though there is no structural improvements in the bowel. A gluten-free diet prohibits wheat, rye, oats, and their products such as bread, buns, cakes, and biscuits, as well as foods such as gravies and soups which have wheat flour added to them.	**Malabsorption syndrome**

Malacia	Softening of part of an organ.
Malaise	Listlessness, tiredness, irritability, depression, distress, and general feeling of illness; often a forerunner of some feverish infection.
Malar	Of or relating to the cheek; the cheekbone; the *zygoma*.
Malaria	An infection characterized by chills and intermittent or remitting fever, caused by parasites transmitted to man by the bites of mosquitoes.
Mal de mer	Seasickness; a form of MOTION SICKNESS.
Male climacteric	An indefinite state in elderly men, analogous to the menopause in women but without a clearcut sign comparable to cessation of menstruation which marks the female climacteric. Some physical changes occur with age as the hormone output of the sex glands diminishes; it may be difficult to separate physical factors from psychological reactions to fears, worries, boring environment, retirement, decreased sexual functions and opportunity, unrecognized illness, depression, apprehensive brooding on the passage of time. Vague symptons self-attributed to the male climacteric call for a visit to the doctor, who may decide that hormone treatment is worth a trial, or may find some condition that requires quite different treatment. Symptons associated with diminished male hormone production (restorable to normal maintenance levels by replacement therapy) are decreased sexual potential, irritability, depression, lack of concentration, and diminished growth of beard and body hair.
Malignant	Life threatening; the usual medical meaning is cancerous.
Malingering	The feigning of illness. The motive may be to avoid work, collect damages, or gain sympathy. The deception can usually be exposed by tests and observations not recognized or understood by the malingerer.
Mallet finger	A dislocation of the end joint of a finger, which cannot be

lifted, due to rupture or tearing of a tendon by a direct blow from a cricket ball or other object upon the end or back of the finger.

Malleus

One of the three tiny bones (*ossicles*) of the middle ear which amplify vibrations of the eardrum and conduct them to the inner ear. Malleus means 'hammer'; the handle of the hammer, attached to the eardrum, amplifies vibrations which are transmitted to the adjacent anvil-bone.

Malocclusion

Inharmonious meeting of the upper and lower teeth; poor bite; bad alignment of teeth and jaws.

Malpresentation

Any position of the fetus in the birth outlet other than the normal head-down position at childbirth; for example, breech, forehead, or foot presentation.

Malta fever

See BRUCELLOSIS

Mammography

X-rays of the breast, several views are taken, to improve accuracy in detecting very small lesions.

Mammoplasty

Plastic surgery for the breast, especially an operation to correct sagging breasts. It is performed by excising tissue and fixing the glands in their normal position.

Mandible

The lower jawbone.

Manic-depressive psychosis

A form of mental illness. It is characterized by swings from intense elation and hyperactivity to deep depression; between swings the patient may act quite normally. In the manic phase, the patient is enormously optimistic, overtalkative, physically busy, always on the go; his thoughts skip wildly from one subject to another; he is excited by grandiose projects. In the depressive phase, he may be hopelessly discouraged, have feelings of utter worthlessness, hear voices which nag him, and may have difficulty in performing the simplest mental and physical tasks.

Manubrium

The uppermost part of the breastbone.

Marasmus	Wasting and emaciation of infants; causes are various.
March fracture	Painful swelling and fracture of bones of the foot, not produced by acute injury but by excessive strain, as in marching.
Marfan's syndrome	A rare hereditary disorder, characterized by unusual flexibility of joints, disproportionately long legs, flabby tissues, funnel chest or pigeon breast, spider fingers, flat foot, displacement of the lens of the eye, and heart defects. The fundamental defect appears to be in connective tissue which breaks down or fails to produce normal amounts of fibres to support body structures.
Marginal ulcer	A peptic ulcer occuring at the junction where the stomach and jejunum have been surgically united.
Marie-Strumpell disease (*ankylosing spondylitis*)	A progressive disease of joints of the spine, different from rheumatoid arthritis.
Marrow	Soft material which fills the cavities of bones. Formation of blood cells takes place in the *red marrow* of certain bones of adults and of all bones in early life. *Yellow marrow* is fatty material which does not perform any blood-making function.
Masseter	A muscle that moves the lower jaw in chewing.
Mastectomy	Surgical removal of the breast, usually because of cancer.
Mastitis	Inflammation of the breasts, from bacterial infection or other causes. The most common disease of the female breasts is *chronic mastitis*; the breasts contain nodules and small cysts of rubbery consistency, usually painful. A lump in the breast is not necessarily cancer, but it is imperative to consult a doctor to determine its nature.
Mastodynia	Pain in the breast.
Mastoid	Refers to mastoid air cells which surround the middle ear.

Infection reaching these cells from the middle ear may require *mastoidectomy*, surgical removal of affected cells.

Substances used in medicine, and the science concerned with the origin, preparation, dosage and administration, and actions of the substances. **Materia medica**

The upper jawbone. **Maxilla**

A pyramid-shaped cavity, largest of the nasal sinuses, located in the front of the upper jaw on each side of the nose. Also called *antrum*. The floor of the cavity is close to the root of the eye-tooth. **Maxillary sinus**

An infectious disease caused by a virus. Although most children recover from a natural attack of measles without suffering serious after-effects, the disease can be treacherous. It can lead to ENCEPHALITIS and mental retardation. Immunizing vaccines make it unnecessary for any child to be exposed to such risk. One injection of live-virus measles vaccine gives long-lasting, probably lifetime immunity. **Measles** (*rubeola*)

An opening or passage, such as the external opening of the urethra. **Meatus**

A pouch opening from the small intestine, a blind tube two to five inches long. It is normally obliterated in the course of fetal development, but in some people it remains as a vestigial remnant. It may become inflamed and cause symptons resembling appendicitis. **Meckel's diverticulum**

Pasty, greenish material which fills the intestines of the fetus before birth and forms the first bowel movement of the newborn. *Meconium ileus*, obstruction of the intestines by viscid meconium, is the earliest manifestation of *cystic fibrosis*. **Meconium**

The space in the middle of the chest between lungs, breastbone, and spine, containing the heart, great blood vessels, oesophagus, windpipe, and associated structures. **Mediastinum**

Medical genetics

The science concerned with associations of heredity with defects and disease.

Medulla

The inside parts of certain organs, such as glands and bones, as distinguished from the cortex or surface layer of the organ. The word also means marrow-like.

Medulla oblongata

The lowest part of the brain, where it merges with the spinal cord. It resembles a bulb at the end of the spinal cord. It contains vital nerve centres which control such functions as heart action, breathing, and swallowing.

Megacolon

Gigantic colon. In a congenital form known as *Hirschsprung's disease*, the colon lacks nerve cells necessary for its emptying. The symptoms are greatly enlarged abdomen and intractable constipation; days may go by without a bowel movement. An acquired type of megacolon usually has a psychological basis; the child refuses to have a bowel movement and the rectum and colon become greatly distended from the mass of retained faeces.

Megakaryocyte

A giant cell of the bone marrow. Fragments of this cell are blood PLATELETS essential for normal coagulation of blood.

Meibomian glands

Sebaceous glands of the eye-lid, subject to infection (*stye*) and obstruction (CHALAZION).

Melaena

Black, tarry stools discoloured by the presence of blood altered in the intestinal tract, as in bleeding from the stomach or intestines. Melaena of the newborn occasionally occurs from seepage of blood into the alimentary tract and is rarely a symptom of disease. Otherwise, passage of tarry stools calls for medical investigation.

Melanin

A brown to black pigment which is a factor in skin colour. It is derived from an AMINO ACID, tyrosine, through the action of an enzyme; if the enzyme is missing the person is an albino. Its production is stimulated by a hormone of the pituitary gland. Suntan, freckles, and flat brown spots on the skin of elderly people are examples of melanin deposits.

A dark mole coloured by melanin granules. The word often means *malignant melanoma*, a dangerous form of cancer, arising from pigment-producing cells. Blue or black moles may be removed as a preventive measure. Moles that darken or increase in size or appear after the age of 30 can be dangerous and should be removed.

Melanoma

A thin layer of tissue which lines a part, separates cavities, or connects adjacent structures.

Membrane

The time of the first occurrence of menstruation. The periods may be irregular while the menstrual cycle is becoming established. The average age at onset of menses is eleven to thirteen years; variations of a year on either side of the average are not unusual. If menstruation is not established before or shortly after the sixteenth year, the cause should be investigated.

Menarche

Membranes which cover the brain and spinal cord.

Meninges

Inflammation of the MENINGES.

Meningitis

Cessation of menses; the milestone which marks the end of a woman's reproductive years. The average age at menopause is 48 years, but it is not unusual for women to continue to menstruate up to or beyond 50 years of age. At menopause, menstruation may cease abruptly, or there may be a gradual increase in the number of days between menstrual periods over a year or two. The final menstrual cycles are usually *anovulatory* – that is, no egg cells are produced by the ovaries. Many cycles which occur long before the menopause are probably anovulatory, but this cannot be relied on as assurance against conception. The average menstrual life span is about 33 years, during which a mature egg cell is released from the ovaries every month. Over the years fewer and fewer cells which develop into ova remain in the ovaries. Along with the dwindling numbers of such there is a progressive decrease in production of ovarian hormones. Hot flushes and other symptoms of the menopause reflect this decline. Most women adjust to the menopause with little difficulty. A few have to seek medical attention for symptoms which are likely to be more

Menopause

annoying than incapacitating. However, symptoms occuring at this time may be wrongly blamed on the change of life and should be investigated to determine the cause, which may be quite unrelated to the menopause.

Menorrhagia

Excessive menstrual bleeding.

Mental subnormality

Mental subnormality is categorized in three main groups; broadly speaking, a child with an IQ between 70 and 50 is classed as *educationally subnormal*, and a child with an IQ of 50 or below may be classed as *mentally retarded* or *severely mentally retarded*. Children in the last two categories can never live without constant supervision, but the educationally subnormal may be expected to undertake some protected occupation and might live semi-independently, for example in supervised lodgings with meals provided.

Mesentery

The flat, fan-shaped sheet of tissue which carries nerves and blood vessels and supports the intestine, from the handle of the fan attached to the back wall of the abdomen. The arrangement allows considerable freedom of intestinal movement within the abdomen.

Mesomorph

See SOMATOTYPE.

Metabolism

The sum total of all the chemical activities by which life processes are organized and maintained; the breakdown and build-up of complex substances by body cells, assimilation of nutrients, and transformations which make energy available to the living organism. *Basal metabolism* is the minimal amount of heat (energy) needed to sustain activities when the body is in a state of complete rest.

Metaplasia

Alteration of a cell to an abnormal type.

Metastasis

Spread of disease from one part of the body to an unconnected part, by transfer of cells or organisms by blood and lymph channels. Ability to metastasize is characteristic of invasive cancer

Foot pain in the instep area, usually due to weakness of muscles and ill-fitting shoes.	**Metatarsalgia**
The five long bones of the foot, overlying the longitudinal arch, between toe joints and heel.	**Metatarsals**
Distension of stomach or intestines with gases.	**Meteorism**
Inflammation of the uterus.	**Metritis**
Abnormal bleeding from the uterus at times other than the menstrual period.	**Metrorrhagia**
An instrument which cuts extremely thin slices of tissue which are placed on slides, stained, and studied by pathologists.	**Microtome**
The act of passing urine.	**Micturition**
The air-filled cavity between the eardrum and the inner ear. It contains the chain of three tiny bones over which sound vibrations are conducted.	**Middle ear**
Prickly heat, heat rash. Obstruction of sweat glands traps sweat under the skin, producing small blisters. The condition disappears when the stimulus to sweating is removed, as by a cool environment.	**Miliaria**
A form of THROMBOPHLEBITIS which occasionally occurs a week or two after childbirth. The affected leg swells and the tense skin has a white appearance, hence the name. Getting out of bed and moving around soon after delivery helps to prevent clot formation in veins. There is very little risk of EMBOLISM in this condition.	**Milk leg**
Extra breasts or nipples are congenital anomalies that occur occasionally in men and women. Supernumerary nipples with little or no underlying breast tissue are more common than miniature out-of-place breasts. In some instances, superfluous breasts of women may attain considerable size and even produce milk. The most frequent site of accessory breasts is	**Milk line**

about three inches below the normal pair, but they may occur anywhere along an imaginary line running from the armpit to the groin on either side. This is called the milk line, and marks the course of structures which permit the development of multiple breasts in mammals other than man. Development of accessory breasts along this line is determined early in fetal life.

Milk teeth

Baby teeth; the twenty teeth which are shed when the permanent teeth erupt.

Miller-Abbott tube

A double-channelled tube for insertion through the nose into the stomach to relieve distension of the small bowel. One channel has a small balloon at the end which is inflated in the stomach; peristaltic movements carry the tube farther down. Intestinal contents are withdrawn through the other channel.

Mineralocorticoids

Hormones of the cortex of the adrenal gland which regulate salt and water balance.

Miscarriage

Expulsion of the fetus before it is capable of independent life. See ABORTION.

Mitochondria

Minute sausage-shaped particles in both cells, which contain the chemical machinery for generating energy. A typical mitochondrion has an outside membrane and numerous connecting interfolds. The outer membrane extracts energy from molecules derived from food and moves it to inner membranes which make ATP (*adenosine triphosphate*), the form of energy that keeps life processes going.

Mitral valve

The valve on the left side of the heart which admits oxygenated blood to the main pumping chamber, the left ventricle. The valve has two peaked flaps shaped somewhat like a bishop's mitre. The valve may be damaged by rheumatic fever so that it leaks, or is scarred and thickened and cannot open widely enough.

Mittelschmerz

A sign of OVULATION; lower abdominal pain produced by

escape of blood into the peritoneal cavity as a result of ovulation, about midway in the menstrual cycle. The nature of the pain is usually identified by absence of any signs of pelvic disease and onset of menses about fourteen days later.

See HYDATIDIFORM MOLE.	**Molar pregnancy**

A contagious viral infection of the skin, producing yellowish pimples containing cheesy material.	**Molluscum contagiosum**

A bluish spot or spots in the region of the lower back, seen in some newborn infants. The congenital spots usually disappear by the fourth or fifth year. Not related to MONGOLISM.	**Mongolian spot**

A congenital abnormality. Mongol babies tend to have upward slanting eyes, broad face, flattened skull, short hands, feet, and trunk, stubby nose, and lax limbs. The average mongol seldom achieves a mental capacity beyond that of a three to seven-year-old child, but is often lively and lovable. Life expectancy is not great. Placement in an institution is often recommended, especially if there are other children in the family. Mongolism results from a specific defect in CHROMO-SOMES, called *trisomy*. One set of chromosomes is not a normal pair, but a triplet. The extra mongolism chromosome causes defects of physical and mental development. The mongoloid child has 47 instead of the normal complement of 46 chromosomes. The parents are in no way responsible for this accident, which occurs sporadically. The older the mother, the greater the risk.	**Mongolism** (*Down's syndrome*)

A type of large white blood cell with a single central mass or nucleus. *Infectious mononcleosis* gets its name from an excess of such cells, arising from infection.	**Monocyte**

A substance used to enhance the flavours of foods. It is a concentrated source of sodium and would not be permitted in diets in which sodium intake must be kept low.	**Monosodium glutamate**

Developed from a single fertilized egg, as identical twins.	**Monozygotic**

Mons veneris

The rounded prominence of fatty tissue above the external female sex organs.

Morning sickness

The nausea or vomiting of pregnancy. Nausea and vomiting usually occur around breakfast time, then subside, only to recur the next morning. The sympton usually persists for two or three weeks and clears up without treatment. About 50 per cent of pregnant women experience morning sickness. A more serious form of vomiting of pregnancy (*hyperemesis gravidarum*) may go on for weeks, produce serious weight loss, and require medical treatment or a period in hospital.

Morphinism

Addiction to morphine.

Motion sickness

Nausea and vomiting induced by forms of motion which rotate the head simultaneously in more than one plane (sea sickness, car sickness, train sickness, air sickness). The trouble originates in the labyrinth of the ear where the organs of equilibrium are located. Confusing impulses reach the vomiting centre in the brain. Motion sickness may sometimes be prevented or minimized by not overeating or overdrinking; by lying down; by taking a position where motion is least exaggerated; by not reading or looking out of a car window or watching a rolling horizon from a boat. A number of drugs help to prevent or lessen motion sickness.

Mountain sickness

A temporary condition brought on by diminished amounts of oxygen in the air at high altitudes. Persons who live at high altitudes adapt to the thin air; their red corpuscles increase in number. Acute mountain sickness is most likely to affect persons who are suddenly transported to high altitudes and do strenuous work. The symptoms usually abate in a few days to a week.

Mouth breathing

The habit of breathing through the mouth instead of the nose has a drying action on the mouth tissues, which become inflamed, sometimes swollen and painful. Mouth breathers usually have a high incidence of colds and upper respiratory infections because they do not have the normal protection of the filtering, warming, air-conditioning functions of the nose.

Physical factors may encourage mouth breathing. Children with narrow nasal passages, easily stuffed up by a minor cold, tend to breathe through the mouth. Enlarged adenoid or tonsil tissue, which normally grows in excess up to about ten years of age and then diminishes, may obstruct the airway and force the child to breathe through the mouth, which can easily become a habit. A doctor or dentist can diagnose mouth breathing easily, determine if there is a physical cause, and help a child to overcome a harmful habit with unpleasant consequences.

Mouth ulcers
(*aphthous ulcers*)

Little blisters on membranes of the mouth and cheeks which break and leave open sores. The painful ulcers usually heal spontaneously in a week or so but attacks may be recurrent. It is no longer thought that mouth ulcers are caused by viruses (the sores may appear at the same time as cold sores or fever blisters which are caused by herpes simplex virus). A bacterial cause is suspected. Persons who have repeated or continuous crops of mouth ulcers may be allergic to some substance in the bacterium's make-up. The organism is sensitive to tetracycline an antibiotic; oral suspensions of the drug held in the mouth for two minutes and then swallowed (four times daily) shorten the healing time but do not prevent recurrences.

Mucous colitis

Not an organic disease, but the over-reaction of an easily irritated colon to various stimuli such as emotions or foods. Passage of mucus with bowel movements is harmless.

Mucous membrane

Mucus-secreting tissue lining the inner walls of body cavities and passages which contain or may contain a certain amount of air and hence could dry out if not moistened. Mucous membranes are similar in general design but perform somewhat different functions in various parts of the body. Mucous membranes of the nose warm and moisten air before it reaches the lungs. Membranes of the windpipe are equipped with fine hairlike processes which sweep a thin film of mucus containing trapped particles of dust and dirt outwards from the lungs. Membranes of the stomach have special glands concerned with digestion; the membrane of the uterus undergoes periodic changes of engorgement and recession linked with the menstrual cycle.

Mucus

Watery material secreted by mucous membranes, normally thin and unobtrusive, profuse in the presence of head colds, and subject to thickening and stickiness if its water becomes greatly reduced.

Multipara

A woman who has previously given birth to several children.

Multiple births

The statistical chance of a mother's giving birth to twins is about one in 90 and the odds against triplets, quadruplets, or quintuplets are very much greater. Twins are more frequent in countries with high birth rates and more frequent among coloured than white people. There is some tendency for fraternal (two-egg) twins to run in families. Women under the age of twenty have the lowest incidence of twins and women between 35 and 39 have the highest. Likelihood of having twins is greater if a woman has already borne children and greater yet if any of those children were twins. Treatment with gonadotrophin hormones to stimulate fertility seems to increase the likelihood of multiple births.

Mummification

Drying and shrivelling of tissue to a mummy-like mass, a result of dry GANGRENE

Mumps vaccine

It is of the attenuated live virus type (see VACCINE) which gives lasting immunity.

Muscae volitantes

Spots and threads before the eyes; floating specks. This common condition increases with age, and is not of serious significance.

Muscle

About half the body's weight is muscle, a remarkable tissue which has the ability to contract and shorten its length. It is about 80 per cent water and most of the rest is protein. We have three types of muscle, different in function and visibly different under a microscope. Muscles we are most aware of are the ones that move our bones and make it possible to chew, walk, and execute all manner of movements. This type is called *striped, voluntary,* or *skeletal* muscle. It has dark and light crossbands giving a striped appearance. Voluntary muscles move when we will them to; their ends are connected to the parts they move. (The only voluntary muscle that is not attached at both ends is the tongue.) Another type of muscle is called *smooth, visceral,* or *involuntary,* It has no cross-striping. It is present in the walls of the digestive tract, blood vessels, bladder, uterus, lungs, and other tissues, where it works without our conscious command. The pupil of the eye changes its size involuntarily; we are propelled into the world by the involuntary contractions of smooth uterine muscles. A third type of muscle is unique. It constitutes the heart muscle (*myocardium*). It is a firm network of fibres connected to one another to function as a unit. Muscle contraction requires energy, produces heat, and is responsible for most of the body temperature. Even when resting , muscles are in a constant state of mild contraction (*tonus*). *Muscle cramps* result from continuous nerve impulses which keep a muscle in a painful state of contraction. A pulled muscle results from tearing or stretching by some massive effort. Exercise increases the size of muscles by enlarging individual cells, not by adding more cells.

Mutation

A change in the hereditary material of an organism, producing a change in some characteristic of the organism; especially, alteration of the character of a GENE. Mutations may occur spontaneously or they may be induced by some external stimulus, such as irradiation.

Myasthenia gravis

A chronic disease characterized by rapid fatigue of certain muscles, with prolonged time of recovery of function. The muscles of the eyes and throat are most often affected, producing such symptons as inability to raise the eyelids, difficulties of swallowing and talking, loss of chewing power, impairment of breathing. The muscles do not waste away. It is thought that the patient lacks some chemical concerned with nerve transmission. A drug called *neostigmine* acts at nerve and muscle fibre junctions to restore considerable muscle power quite rapidly. Many myasthenia gravis patients have an enlarged *thymus gland* or tumours of the thymus. X-ray treatment or surgical removal of the gland has produced some remissions, but results of these treatments for individual patients are not predictable.

Mycetoma	See MADURA FOOT.
Mycoses	Infections caused by fungi.
Myelin	White fatty material which covers most nerve AXONS, in the manner of insulation around an electric wire; it is essential to proper transmission of nerve impulses. Degeneration or disappearance of the myelin sheath is the characteristic lesion of *demyelinating disease*.
Myelitis	Inflammation of the spinal cord or bone marrow. *Poliomyelitis* is inflammation of grey matter of the cord.
Myelogram	An X-ray film of the spinal canal made after injecting a contrast medium opaque to X-rays.
Myeloma, *multiple*	Malignant tumours of the bone marrow.
Myiasis	Infestation with larvae of flies which may develop in the skin, eyes, ear, or nose, and in wounds.
Myocarditis	Inflammation of the heart muscle.
Myocardium	The heart muscle; a highly specialized, cross-layered, very powerful involuntary muscle. Shutting off the blood supply to a portion of the muscle, as in coronary thrombosis, results in local death of tissue (*infarction*), a common sequel to heart attack.
Myocyte	A muscle cell.
Myoglobin	A form of HAEMOGLOBIN, slightly different from that of the blood, which is present in muscles and serves as a short-term source of oxygen to tide muscle fibres from one contraction to another.
Myoma	A tumour composed of muscle elements; it is a common

benign tumour of the uterus.

The muscle of the uterus.	**Myometrium**
Any disease of muscle.	**Myopathy**
Shortsightedness.	**Myopia**
Inflammation of muscle.	**Myositis**
Inflammation of the eardrum.	**Myringitis**
Surgical repair of a damaged eardrum.	**Myringoplasty**
Incision of the eardrum ro relieve pressure of pus behind it.	**Myringotomy**
Thyroid deficiency, *hypothyroidism* in adults. Congenital thyroid deficiency in children is known as *cretinism*. The patient with untreated mysoedema has dry, thick, puffy skin, thinning hair, low metabolism, is sensitive to cold, thick of speech, and mentally sluggish.	**Myxoedema**
A tumour derived from connective tissue.	**Myxoma**

N

A local area of pigmentaton or elevation of the skin; a mole, a birthmark.	**Naevus**
An ammonia burn resulting from breakdown of urine.	**Nappy rash**
Self-love, undue admiration of one's own body; a psychological term indicating self-admiration fixed at a level appropriate to infants but not to adults.	**Narcissism**
Irresistable attacks of sleep, often with transient muscular weakness. Attacks occur during normal waking hours, not only under conditions conducive to drowsiness – after a heavy meal, during a dull lecture, in a train – but in inappropriate and even hazardous circumstances as in driving a car. The affected person usually sleeps a few minutes, wakes refreshed, but may fall asleep again in a short time. The sleep does not differ from normal sleep except in its untimeliness; there are no signs of disease or physical abnormality. Treatment with drugs is usually successful in warding off attacks of sleepiness during the day.	**Narcolepsy**
A state of deep sleep, unconsciousness, and insensibility to pain. *Narcotics* are drugs that produce such effects. Such drugs are very important in medicine, but if misused can lead to drug addiction.	**Narcosis**
The top part of the throat, behind the nasal cavity.	**Nasopharynx**
See MORNING SICKNESS.	**Nausea of pregnancy**
The point closest to the eye where an object, such as small print, is seen distinctly, normally 25cm (10 in).	**Nearpoint**
Autopsy; a postmortem examination.	**Necropsy**
Death of a localized portion of tissue surrounded by living tissue.	**Necrosis**
Round or oval particles in certain cells of animals dead of *rabies*. Their presence is proof that the animal had rabies.	**Negri bodies**

Neisserian infection	Usually means infection with gonorrhoea germs. *Neisseria gonorrhoea*.
Neonatal	Newborn; the first two or three days of life.
Neoplasm	Any abnormal new growth; a tumour which may be malignant or benign. Neoplastic disease is a common term for cancer.
Nephrectomy	Surgical removal of a kidney.
Nephritis	Inflammation of the kidney.
Nephrolith	Kidney stone.
Nephroma	Malignant tumour of the cortex of the kidney.
Nephron	The urine-forming unit of the kidney. It consists of a double-walled cup-shaped structure(*Bowman's capsule*) within which a tuft of tiny blood vessels (*the glomerulus*) exudes blood constituents which pass as a dilute filtrate into the tubule of the capsule. Most of the water and some essential materials in the filtrate are reabsorbed and the remainder is concentrated as urine.
Nephrosclerosis	Nephritis due to hardening of kidney blood vessels.
Nephrosis	Degeneration of the kidney without signs of inflammation; usually refers to nephrotic disease of children.
Nephrotoxic	Poisonous to the kidneys.
Nerve	Any of the cordlike bundles of fibres, composed of microscopic neutrons, along which nerve impulses travel.
Nerve deafness	Impairment of hearing from partial or complete failure of the auditory nerves to transmit impulses to the brain.
Nettle rash (*urticaria*)	Whitish, intensely itching elevations of the skin; weals, resembling mosquito bites and usually larger, sometimes covering patches as large as the palm. An attack may be a solitary event,

never again experienced, subsiding in a few days, but in some instances nettle rash is repeated and persistent. Frequently the condition is an allergic reaction to certain foods (strawberries, shellfish, etc.), to drugs, to cold, to heat, or to sunlight.

Severe pain in a nerve or along its course, with demonstrable change in the structure of the nerve. The pain is typically sharp, stabbing, and severe, though short-lasting.	**Neuralgia**
A somewhat unfashionable term for a state of great fatigability, listlessness, aches and pains, once attributed to depletion or exhaustion of nerve centres, but without any demonstrable abnormality of the nervous system. Neurasthenic symptoms may have some organic cause and medical examination may disclose some treatable condition quite unrelated to nerves. If not, the label neurasthenia indicates a functional disorder with a psychological basis.	**Neurasthenia**
Inflammation of a nerve, due to infection, toxins, compression, or other causes.	**Neuritis**
A chronic skin condition of unknown cause, not related to infection or allergy. It occurs most frequently in nervous women and may have a neurotic basis. Itchy patches of thickened skin (see LICHENIFICATION) occur especially on the neck, the inner surface of the elbows, and the backs of the knees. Treatment to relieve itching and discourage rubbing of the skin helps to alleviate the condition.	**Neurodermatitis**
A condition of multiple tumours in the skin along nerve pathways. The tumours, mainly composed of fibrous material, tend to increase in size and number. The growths are not cancerous, but very rarely may undergo malignant transformation. Sometimes the tumours can be removed surgically, often permanently, although in some cases they have a tendency to recur. The disorder is thought to be hereditary.	**Neurofibromatosis**
Of nervous origin.	**Neurogenic**
The complete nerve cell, including the cell body, *dendrites*	**Neuron**

which bring incoming impulses to the body, and the *axon* which carries impulses away from it.

Neuropsychiatry	The medical specialty concerned with both nervous and mental disorders and their overlap.
Neurosis	See PSYCHONEUROSIS.
Neurosurgery	The surgery of the central nervous syetm.
Neurosyphilis	A late stage of syphilis affecting the central nervous system.
Neutrophil	A type of white blood cell stainable by neutral dyes. *Neutropenia* is scarcity of such cells in the blood.
Nictitation	Blinking.
Nidation	Implantation of a fertilized egg in the uterus.
Nidus	A nest; a point of origin or focus.
Nieman-Pick disease	A rare hereditary condition occuring almost exclusively in children of Jewish families. It is a disorder of LIPID metabolism (inability to handle fatlike substances) which progresses to anaemia, emaciation, mental retardation, blindness, and deafness. Affected children rarely survive their second year. There is no treatment. The disease is inherited as a recessive trait.
Nightblindness (*nyctalopia*)	Imperfect vision at night or in dim light; reduced dark adaptation. The symptom may result from deficiency of vitamin A, which is necessary for regeneration of nerve cells of the retina (rods). These do most of the seeing when light is poor. Certain diseases of the retina can also cause nightblindness.
Nitrogen balance	An expression of the body's PROTEIN balance, determined by measurements of its nitrogen constituents. If nitrogen intake exceeds excretion, the balance is positive. Excessive retention of nitrogen may indicate kidney disease or other conditions. Negative nitrogen balance may indicate inadequate dietary protein, excessive loss of protein due to toxic goitre, burns,

draining wounds, and so on, impaired absorption of protein, or defective metabolism of protein as in some liver diseases.

A drug, derived from mustard gas, used to destroy malignant cells in lymphomatous diseases.   **Nitrogen mustard**

Laughing gas; an inhalant for producing brief anaesthesia, as for tooth extraction.   **Nitrous oxide**

Excessive urination at night.   **Nocturia**

A small protuberance, swelling, rounded knob, knot of cells. A *nodule* is a small node.   **Node**

Enlargement of the thyroid gland, characterized by lumpy masses in the gland.   **Nodular goitre**

Incapable of living.   **Nonviable**

Normal blood pressure.   **Normotension**

Of or relating to a hospital.   **Nosocomial**

Of or relating to, or in the region of, the nape of the neck.   **Nuchal**

Radioisotopes of an element decay spontaneously, ultimately reverting to a stable atom, and in the process give off energy in the form of radiation which is detectable by sensitive devices. Thus substances marked or labelled with radio-isotopes (for example, radioactive iodine, phosphorus, chromium) can be followed in their course through the body, giving information about the chemical process of life. Drugs can be marked in this way to gain new knowledge of how they work. Recently developed *scintillation cameras* translate iso-tope emissions into dots on film, giving a pattern of radiation within a patient's body. Certain tissues are selective for certain elements; the thyroid gland, for instance, takes up iodine. Radioisotopes which tend to concentrate in such tissues may be given in larger doses with the object of destroying or reducing the functioning of cells. Diagnostically, radioisotopes   **Nuclear medicine** help to measure the functional abilities of certain tissues, are useful in evaluating some blood disorders, and in locating and marking the boundaries of tumours.

Nucleus

The rounded central body of a cell, surrounded by cytoplasm. It contains the CHROMOSOMES and mechanisms of cell division and heredity.

Nullipara

A woman who has never born a child.

Nummular eczema

Dry skin with coin-shaped plaques on the back of hands and outer surfaces of the arms, legs, and thighs.

Nyctalopia

See NIGHT BLINDNESS.

Nymphomania

EXCESSIVE sexual desire in a woman.

Nystagmus

Involuntary, rhythmic oscillation of the eyeballs, horizontal, vertical, or rotatory. Most people experience nystagmus if the body is whirled to produce dizziness and an attempt is made to fix the gaze on a stationary object. Simple forms of nystagmus can result from eye strain or refractive errors. Nystagmus may be a sympton of inner ear disturbance or disorder of the nervous system.

O

Two curved flat blades (right and left) which are separately placed with great care around the head of the fetus in the birth passage; the handles are then interlocked. Used to assist extraction of the baby in difficult deliveries.	**Obstetric forceps**
A doctor specializing in the care of pregnant women.	**Obstetrician**
The back part of the head.	**Occiput**
Closure or shutting off, as of a blood vessel; also, the meeting position of upper and lower teeth when closed.	**Occlusion**
Hidden, not evident to the naked eye; as, occult blood in faeces.	**Occult**
Of or relating to the eye.	**Ocular**
Disharmony of muscles which move the eyeball. Associated with such conditions as squint, poor fusion of images, amblyopia.	**Ocular muscle imbalance**
Same as OPHTHALMOLOGIST.	**Oculist**
Excessive accumulation of fluid in blood cavities and spaces around cells. The fluid produces swelling of waterlogged tissues. Oedema is not a disease but a symptom of varying importance. The waterlogging may be mild and localized, such as the puffiness around a bruise or a slight swelling of the ankles after standing all day, or it may distend almost all the body like a balloon. The underlying cause may be trivial, as in PREMENSTRUAL TENSION, or serious. Pitting oedema, the kind which leaves a little pit or depression when pressed, is often associated with heart or kidney disorders. Oedema results from some disturbance of the mechanisms of fluid exchange in the body, of which there are many causes; salt and water retention by the kidneys (see ELECTROLYTES), congestive heart failure, allergy, protein deficiency, obstruction of lymphatic drainage (see LYMPHOEDEMA), inflammation, injury, liver and kidney disease, tumours. Modern diuretic drugs which increase the output of urine and dispose of excess fluid are	**Oedema**

helpful in the management of oedema while the underlying disease is treated.

Oesophagitis	Inflammation of the lining of the oesophagus.
Oesophagus	The gullet; the muscular tube through which swallowed food passes into the stomach by muscular action.
Oestrogen	A general term for female sex hormones.
Oil pneumonia	See ASPIRATION PNEUMONIA.
Olecranon	A curved part of one of the forearm bones (*ulna*) at the elbow end. It is what we lean on when we rest an elbow on a table.
Olfactory bulb	A structure just above the thin bone which separates the top of the nasal cavity from the brain. It receives nerve fibres that pass upwards through small holes in the bone from the nose.
Oligomenorrhoea	Scanty menstrual flow, or abnormally long time between menstrual periods.
Oligophrenia	Mental deficiency, feeblemindedness.
Oligospermia	Abnormally few SPERMATOZOA in the semen.
Oliguria	Scanty secretion of urine; abnormal infrequency of urination.
Omentum	A layer of tissue, a fold of the peritoneum, that hangs from the stomach and transverse colon and covers the underlying organs like an apron. It forms a fat pad on the front of the abdomen, sometimes conspicuously thick.
Onchocerciasis	A form of FILARIASIS occurring in tropical areas. Infection with threadlike worms produces tumours in the skin and sometimes blinding disease of the eyes.

O

The science of tumours, new growths.	**Oncology**
Inflammation of the bed of a nail, often resulting in loss of the nail.	**Onychia**
Inflammation of the eye, especially with involvement of the conjunctiva.	**Ophthalmia**
A doctor who specializes in medical and surgical care of the eyes.	**Ophthalmologist**
An instrument which gives a view of structures inside the eye.	**Ophthalmoscope**
Narcotics from or related to opium; for example, morphine, heroin, codeine, paregoric, laudanum. In a broad sense the word applies to any sense-dulling, stupor-inducing drug.	**Opiates**
A position in the body in which the head and lower legs are bent backwards and the trunk arched forwards, due to convulsive spasm of muscles of the back, such as in strychnine poisoning.	**Opisthotonos**
Irreversible degeneration of optic nerve fibres.	**Optic atrophy**
An arrangement of nerve fibres in which the optic nerves of both eyes cross at a junction near the pituitary gland.	**Optic chiasma**
The area at the back of the eyes where all the nerve fibres of the retina merge with the optic nerve. Because light is not perceived at the point where the optic nerve enters the eye, the area is a normal BLIND SPOT. When using both eyes together, one is unaware of a blind spot.	**Optic disc**
A technician who caries out the prescription of an ophthalmologist for glasses or contact lenses; a manufacturer or designer of optical equipment.	**Optician**
A bundle of a million or so nerve fibres which transmits	**Optic nerve**

impulses from the RETINA to the occipital lobe at the back of the brain where they are transformed into vision.

Oral
Of or relating to the mouth; in the case of medicines, administered by the mouth. (Not to be confused with *aural* – of or relating to the ear.)

Oral contraceptives
STEROID compounds taken by mouth by women to prevent conception; the pill. The tablets contain combinations of oestrogen-progestogen or they may be sequential, furnishing oestrogen alone on certain days of the cycle, followed by combined oestrogen-progestogen. Regularity of dosage is very important.

Orbit
The bony socket that contains the eyeball.

Orchidectomy
Castration; surgical removal of the testicles.

Orchitis
Inflammation of the testicles. It may be a complication of mumps.

Organic disease
Disease that has a physical cause, a lesion, disorder of an organ, as opposed to FUNCTIONAL DISEASE.

Organ of Corti
The centre of the sense of hearing in the inner ear. It contains hairlike cells which oscillate in response to pulsating fluids, stimulating nerve endings which merge into the nerve of hearing that carries impulses to receiving centres in the brain.

Orgasm
The climax of the sexual act, terminating in ejaculation of semen by the male and release of tension in female.

Oriental sore
(*cutaneous leishmaniasis*)
Single or multiple skin ulcers produced by infection with organisms transmitted by sandflies.

Orifice
The opening or outlet of a body cavity or passage.

Ornithosis
(*parrot fever, psittacosis*)
A pneumonia-like disease produced by viruses from infected birds.

O

Tooth straightening; the branch of dental science concerned with prevention and correction of irregularities of the teeth and jaws.	**Orthodontics**
The surgical and medical speciality concerned with correction of deformities, diseases, accidents, and disorders of the body parts that move us about – limbs, bones, joints, muscles, tendons, and so on.	**Orthopaedics**
The need to sit upright in order to breathe comfortably, manifested by persons with congestive heart failure.	**Orthopnoea**
Teaching, training, and exercises for improving the fusion of images from both eyes (as in squint), putting a lazy eye back to work, and generally making visual mechanisms more efficient.	**Orthoptics**
Induced or intensified by standing upright; for example, *orthostatic hypotension*, a lowering of blood pressure brought on by changing from a lying-down to an upright position.	**Orthostatic**
Degeneration of the protuberance on the knee-end of the TIBIA, the long bone of the lower leg. A form of OSTEOCHONDRITIS, occurring most frequently in young persons.	**Osgood-Schlatter disease**
The phenomenon of transfer of materials through a semi-permeable membrane that separates two solutions, or between a solvent and a solution, tending to equalize their concentrations. *Osmotic pressure* is that exerted by the movement of a solvent through a semipermeable membrane into a more concentrated solution on the other side. This pressure is the driving force that causes diffusion of particles in solution to move from one place to another. Walls of living cells are semipermeable membranes and much of the activity of the cells depends upon osmosis.	**Osmosis**
Composed of bone or resembling bone.	**Osseous**
One of the three tiny bones of the middle ear (*malleus, incus, stapes*) which conduct sound vibrations to the inner ear.	**Ossicle**

O

Ossification	The process of forming bone. CARTILAGE is made into bone by the process of ossification. Calcium phosphate is deposited in the cartilage, changing it into bone.
Osteitis	Inflammation of bone.
Osteitis deformans	PAGET'S DISEASE. A chronic process of bone overgrowth, destruction, and new bone formation, ultimately producing deformities. The skull, spine, and weight-bearing bones are most commonly affected.
Osteochondritis	Inflammation of both bone and CARTILAGE. *Osteochondritis dissecans* is a fairly common condition of late adolescence in which there is local death of a section of the joint surface of a bone (usually of the knee) and its overlying cartilage. *Osteochondritis deformans juvenilis* (Perthé's disease) is a degenerative condition of the upper end of the thigh bone in children three to eight years of age, which eventually heals but may leave some permanent deformity of the hip joint.
Osteogenesis imperfecta	A rare hereditary condition of defective formation of bony tissues, resulting in brittle bones which fracture easily.
Osteomalacia	Adult RICKETS; softening of bone, abnormal flexibility, brittleness, loss of calcium salts. Usually due to vitamin D deficiency or impaired absorption of nutrients.
Osteomyelitis	Infection of bone and marrow due to growth of germs within the bone. Infection may reach the bone through the bloodstream or direct injury.
Osteoporosis	Enlargement of canals or spaces in bone, giving a porous thinned appearance. The weakened bone is fragile and may be broken by some minor injury, or may fracture spontaneously. The condition is common in women after the menopause and occurs to some degree in old men.
Osteotome	A surgical instrument used for cutting through bone.
Otalgia	Earache.

Inflammation of the ear. *Otitis externa* is a bacterial or fungal infection of the ear canal. *Otitis media* is an acute or chronic infection of the middle ear.	**Otitis**
Plastic surgery for correction of malformed ears. See PROTRUDING EARS.	**Otoplasty**
A specialist in diseases of the ear, nose, and throat. An *otologist* confines himself to the ear.	**Otorhinolaryngologist**
Chronic discharge from the ear.	**Otorrhoea**
Overgrowth in parts of the middle ear of spongy bone which dampens vibrations, and impairs hearing. This type of hearing loss is often correctible by surgery.	**Otosclerosis**
A patient who comes to a hospital for treatment but does not reside there.	**Outpatient**
A membrane-covered opening to the inner ear, to which the footplate of the STAPES is attached. Sounds conducted by the chain of bones in the middle ear are hammered against the oval window and transmitted to fluids behind it and thence to the inner ear.	**Oval window**
A sac containing fluid or mucoid material arising in the ovary. A cyst with a stem may become twisted and produce sudden severe pain in the lower abdomen.	**Ovarian cyst**
Surgical removal of one or both ovaries, Also called *oophorectomy*.	**Ovariectomy**
Release of a mature egg cell from the follicle in the ovary in which it develops. This is the time during the menstrual cycle when conception can occur. There is no infallible signs of ovulation that a woman can recognize, but there are suggestive signs. Ovulation usually occurs about midway between menstrual periods in a normal menstrual cycle of approximately 28 days. Body temperature tends to rise, though to a small degree, at the time of ovulation. Abdominal pain and a pinkish	**Ovulation**

discharge from the vagina may also occur at the time of ovulation; see INTERMENSTRUAL PAIN, and MITTELSCHMERZ.

Ovum

The female reproductive cell; an egg. The ovum is the largest human cell but is barely discernible by the naked eye. It is about half of the size of the full stop at the end of the sentence. It is a round cell with a clear capsule, and with the consistency of stiff jelly. Like the sperm, the ovum contains only 23 CHROMOSOMES, which at conception pair off with those of the sperm to give the embryo a normal complement of 46 chromosomes. Although the ovum is about 85,000 times larger than the sperm, both contain the same number of GENES. The relatively huge size of the ovum is partly accounted for by its content of nutrient yolk. Only about 400 ova ripen to maturity and are released by ovulation during a woman's reproductive lifetime; of these, only a very few are fertilized.

Oxyhaemoglobin

HAEMOGLOBIN carrying a full load of oxygen; the haemoglobin in bright red arterial blood.

Oxytocin

A hormone of the pituitary gland which stimulates the uterus to contract. It is frequently administered into a vein in order to stimulate labour and ensure effective contractions.

Oxyuriasis

Threadworm or pinworm infection.

Ozaena

A chronic disease of mucous membranes of the nose, giving off a foul-smelling odour or discharge.

A small knot of tissue in the right atrium of the heart which triggers the heartbeat. In certain heart disorders, battery-powered devices connected to the heart can take over the pacemaking function. See CARDIAC PACEMAKER.	**Pacemaker**
Thick-skinned.	**Pachydermatous**
A doctor specializing in the care of children.	**Paediatrician**
Two diseases bear this name. *Paget's disease of the breast* is manifested by thickened, eczema-like scaliness of the area around the nipple, with fissuring, oozing, and destruction of the nipple as the underlying disease (cancer of the central ducts of the breast) advances. The other Paget's disease, also known as *osteitis deformans*, is a chronic disease of bone metabolism. The skull, pelvis, spine, and long bones are especially affected. Calcium and phosphorus are lost from the bones, which become soft and bend easily. Irregular replacement of the minerals causes thickening and deformity. Bone pain, impaired hearing, and muscle cramps are frequent symptoms. The disease progresses slowly and after many years may lead to chronic invalidism.	**Paget's disease**
Primary dysmenorrhoea is characterized by pain, cramps, or mild to severe discomfort occurring at the onset of menstrual periods, in the absence of any organic disorder. Physical exercises may help to banish distress. Any exercise which involves systematic twisting, bending, and extending of the trunk is helpful.	**Painful menstruation**
Limitation of motion and pain about the shoulder may arise from injury, calcium deposits, bursitis, osteoarthritis, diseases of the chest, coronary heart disease. The predominant symptom is severe pain in the shoulder area and inability to raise the arm because of pain and weakness.	**Painful shoulder syndrome**
LEAD POISONING.	**Painter's colic**
Relieving pain, suffering, or distressing symptoms of disease but without any curative action.	**Palliative**

Palpation	A method of obtaining information about a patient's condition by manipulating or feeling a part of the body with the hand.
Palpebral	Of or relating to the eyelid.
Palpitation	Throbbing, pounding, rapid, or fluttering heartbeat, sufficiently out of the ordinary to make the patient aware of it. More often than not the condition is temporary and not of serious importance, but there are many causes and if the symptom is repeated or alarming it should be investigated.
Palsy	Paralysis.
Pancreatitis	Inflammation of the pancreas. It occurs in acute and chronic form.
Pandemic	A super-epidemic, one that occurs on a large scale over a very wide area of a country or of the world.
Panhypopituitarism	Severe loss of function of the anterior pituitary gland.
Panniculus	A layer of fat beneath the skin; the layer on the front of the abdomen sometimes expands the waistline noticeably.
Panophthalmitis	Pus-producing inflammation of all the tissues of the eye, threatening total and permanent blindness.
Papanicolaou smear (*Pap test*)	A screening test for cancer of the cervix and the uterus. Cell scrapings obtained painlessly from the surface of the cervix are spread on glass slides, stained, and examined under a microscope. Detection of cancer cells in the specimen, and confirmation of cancer of the cervix by other diagnostic measures, leads to prompt treatment of a form of cancer which in its early stages is almost invariably curable.
Papilla	A small conical or nipple-shaped elevation, like a pimple. Papillae give the front of the tongue its slightly rough appearance, and orderly lines of papillae projecting into the upper skin layer give us fingerprints.

Noninflammatory swelling of the optic nerve where it enters the eye, due to increased pressure within the skull or interefernce with flow of blood from the veins of the eye. It occurs most frequently in patients with brain tumour, brain abscess, or meningitis; concussion, haemorrhage, or severe hypertension may also be responsible. Vision is good in the early stages, but gradually deteriorates. Treatment depends on detection of the underlying cause.	**Papilloedema** (*choked disc*)
A tumour of lining tissues – skin, mucous membranes, glandular ducts – composed of epithelial cells covering supporting papillae. It is usually benign.	**Papilloma**
A small solid elevation on the skin; a solid pimple containing no pus or fluid.	**Papule**
Surgical puncture of a body cavity to withdraw fluid.	**Paracentesis**
Abnormal sensations of crawling, burning, and tingling of the skin, due to neuritis or lesions of the nervous system.	**Paraesthesia**
A way of heating body parts, especially painful arthritic hands. The hands are dipped into melted paraffin until a thick heat-retaining layer is built up.	**Paraffin wax packs**
Intestinal obstruction resulting from decreased peristaltic activity of the bowel.	**Paralytic ileus**
A form of mental illness characterized by suspiciousness, delusions, feelings of being persecuted, spied upon, or endangered. The patient's delusions are so systematized and seemingly logical that they can be quite convincing to others, especially since the paranoid patient often seems quite sane and reasonable except on one or a few subjects. Mild paranoid trends are not uncommon in suspicious people who think others have it in for them, put obstacles in their way, and are responsible for their failures, but the extreme paranoid, who may do violence to his supposed persecutors, has a severe mental illness.	**Paranoia**

Paraplegia	Paralysis of both legs, usually due to injury or disease of the spinal cord. The bladder and bowels may be paralysed as well as the legs, depending on the controlling part of the nervous system that is injured. Rehabilitation training may restore a good measure of function to the paraplegic patient.
Parathyroid glands	Four pea-size glands embedded superficially on the back and side surfaces of both lobes of the thyroid gland. The glands secrete hormones which maintain a stable concentration of calcium in the blood. Either an excess or deficiency produces mild to serious bodily disturbances.
Paratyphoid	An acute infectious disease which resembles typhoid fever but is less severe. It is caused by Salmonella bacteria transmitted directly or indirectly from the faeces and urine of infected persons.
Parenchyma	The functioning, specialized part of an organ, as distinguished from connective tissue that supports it.
Parenteral	Outside the digestive tract. The word commonly refers to substances given by injection or infusion instead of by mouth.
Paresis	Slight or incomplete paralysis. Also, a term for general paralysis of the insane, resulting from syphilis.
Parietal	Of or relating to the wall of a cavity; especially, the bones of the skull at the top and sides of the head behind the frontal bones.
Parkinson's disease (*parkinsonism*)	A chronic progressive disease of which the chief symptoms are tremor, stiffness, and slowness of movement, resulting from disturbance of a small centre at the base of the brain.
Paronychia	Pus-producing infection of tissues around the nails, caused by yeasts or bacteria. Acute bacterial paronychia is usually treated with antibiotics. Surgical drainage may be necessary. Chronic bacterial paronychia may require prolonged treatment with hot soaking, drainage, and local application of an

antibiotic ointment. During treatment the involved finger or fingers should be kept as dry as possible.

One of the saliva-producing glands, located in the angle of the jaw in front of and below the ear. **Parotid gland**

Inflammation of the parotid gland. Epidemic parotitis is another name for mumps. **Parotitis**

Periodic attacks of extremely rapid beating of the heart, 200 or more beats per minute. Attacks may last only a few seconds or as long as several hours. **Paroxysmal tachycardia**

See PSITTACOSIS. **Parrot fever**

Childbirth. **Parturition**

An indirect method of testing for skin allergies. Serum of the patient is introduced into areas of the skin of another person, and a couple of days later these sites are tested for reactions to suspected allergens. The other person acts as a guinea pig, demonstrating skin reactions to substances to which he himself is not allergic. **Passive transfer**

A method of identifying allergic sensitivities by applying suspected material to the skin. **Patch test**

The kneecap. **Patella**

Blood groups are determined by unvarying laws of heredity. This is the basis of tests for excluding paternity. If a child's red blood cells contain substances which are incompatible with the blood groups of its presumed parents, one of the couple cannot be the father or the other cannot be the mother. A person with AB blood cannot have a child of group O; a person of group O cannot have a child of group AB; a person of group M cannot have a child of group N. Presence or absence of a number of other factors follows the same hereditary rules. The blood factors of the mother, child, and putative father are determined by tests using antiserums and red blood cells **Paternity tests** known to contain A, B, O, M, or N factors. If the factor tested for is present, the red cells clump together; if it is absent they do not. Tests cannot prove that a man *is* the father of a certain child. They prove only that he cannot be, and they cannot always do that because by coincidence his blood may contain the same factors as the actual father. The chance that non-paternity can be proved is a little better than 50 per cent. Only three blood groups (ABO, MN, Rh) are used for medicolegal purposes, but several other factors are known and it is theoretically possible to distinguish 50,000 different blood group combinations. Indeed, it is believed that blood is as individual as fingerprints, and when its chemical markers are more fully revealed it may become possible to determine that a child is the offspring of a particular couple.

Pathogen	An agent causing disease.
Pathogenic	Having the capacity to produce disease. Many bacteria are harmless and even beneficial to man, but the types that cause disease are pathogenic organisms.
Pathology	The science and study of the nature of disease: its processes, effects, causes, manifestations; changes from normal in structure and function. Pathology does not mean disease, but its study. *Pathologists* examine stained cells and tissues, do autopsies, and employ chemical and laboratory methods to assist in diagnosis of disease, identify normal and abnormal structures, and to add to scientific knowledge of disease processes in general.
Pectoral	Of or relating to the chest.
Pedicle graft	A flap of a patient's own skin attached to the body by a stalk or pedicle containing blood vessels that supply nourishment while the flap is taking hold in an area to which it is grafted.
Pediculosis	Infestation with body lice.
Pellagra	A DEFICIENCY DISEASE manifested by rough skin, diarrhoea,

sore mouth and tongue, and sometimes mental disturbance.

Measurement of the dimensions of the body pelvis, usually done to determine whether the outlet of the birth canal is of sufficient size to permit the fetus to be born naturally.	**Pelvimetry**
A basin-shaped cavity, especially that formed by the bones in the hip region. The bony pelvis supports the spinal column, rests on the legs, and contains structures of the lower end of the trunk. The female bony pelvis is slightly different from that of the male. The *kidney pelvis* is a cavity which collects urine from the organ's filtration units and carries it to the ureter and thence to the bladder.	**Pelvis**
An uncommon but serious skin disease manifested by crops of large blisters which rupture and leave raw surfaces.	**Pemphigus**
The major single cause of systemic reactions to drugs is penicillin. Reactions occur in persons previously sensitized to the drug by therapeutic does, or sometimes by indirect contact, as in milk products. The most serious and fortunately the most rare reaction is ANAPHYLAXIS; its most common pattern is acute breathing difficulty, swelling of the larynx threatening suffocation, and profound shock. This reaction occurs within seconds or minutes after administration of penicillin to sensitized patients. Far more common and less serious, but distressing, are skin reactions such as nettle rash and itching. SCRATCH TESTS on persons with no previous history of penicillin sensitization may be performed before administering the drug, but if patients with past histories of penicillin sensitivity are to be tested, emergency treatment facilities should be immediately available.	**Penicillin reactions**
The male sex organ.	**Penis**
A protein-digesting enzyme in the gastric juice. It is active only in an acid environment, which the stomach provides.	**Pepsin**
An ulcer associated with the digestive action of acid juices; it may be located in the stomach or duodenum, or at the site of	**Peptic ulcer**

surgical joining of the stomach and jejunum. The most frequent form is duodenal ulcer.

Percussion

A method of physical diagnosis. Short firm blows are tapped upon a body surface by a finger or small hammer to produce sounds or vibrations. Solid, fluid-filled, tense, empty, or congested organs have different resonances. Percussion is most often applied in examination of the lungs and abdomen.

Perennial allergic rhinitis

A condition similar to hay fever but running a more or less continuous course without seasonal variations.

Perforated eardrum

The eardrum may be punctured by direct injury (never stick hairpins or toothpicks into the ear canal!) or by infections of the middle ear which break through the drum. A punctured eardrum may heal itself, but if not, a route of invasion for infectious material from the outside world is open. A person with a punctured eardrum should not dive or swim or put the head under water because of the danger that infectious material may be forced into internal ear parts. Ear plugs do not give dependable protection. A perforated eardrum can be closed by an operation known as *tympanoplasty*.

Perianal

Situated around the anus.

Pericarditis

Inflammation of the PERICARDIUM from causes such as rheumatic fever or extension of infection from neighbouring parts.

Pericardium

The sac or membrane that encloses the heart. It secretes lubricating fluid that permits free movements of the heart.

Perineum

The area between the anus and scrotum in men, and the anus and the vulva in women.

Periodontal disease

Inflammation of the membranes that cover the roots of the teeth; laymen commonly call it PYORRHOEA.

Periosteum

The membranous covering of nearly all bone surfaces.

Peripheral

At or near an outer surface; for example, peripheral blood

vessels, near skin surfaces.

Wavelike movements of constriction and relaxation which propel materials along the digestive tube. Encircling muscle contracts to squeeze material forward while muscles in front of the material relax; the latter muscles constrict in their turn, and so on.	**Peristalsis**
The strong smooth membrane which lines the abdominal cavity and covers the abdominal organs.	**Peritoneum**
Inflammation of the PERITONEUM; the most frequent cause is a ruptured appendix, but infection can occur from other routes.	**Peritonitis**
Cracks at the side of the mouth, thickened, covered with whitish material. The condition is classically associated with deficiency of a vitamin, riboflavin. Usually the patient has excessive folding of the skin at the corners of the mouth – perhaps congenital, or the result of missing teeth or poorly fitting dentures – and the moist opposing surfaces rub together, resulting in maceration, inflammation, possible infection. The patient licks the cracks, fostering further maceration; spicy or acid foods may be irritating. An ointment may be prescribed, together with appropriate measures to keep the area dry – correction of malocclusion or poorly fitting dentures, abstention from smoking chewing gum, and chewing tobacco.	**Perlèche**
Degeneration of the upper end of the thighbone in young children.	**Perthé's disease**
Whooping cough.	**Pertussis**
One of many devices of metal, rubber, or plastic, of different shapes and sizes, placed in the vagina or the uterus or parts of it to support displaced pelvic structures. Also used of medicated preparations for vaginal insertion.	**Pessary**
Tiny pinpoint haemorrhages in the skin.	**Petechiae**

Petit mal	A form of epileptic attack, consisting of sudden loss of consciousness lasting for only a few seconds.
Pets	See HOUSEHOLD PETS.
pH	Technically, a symbol expressing hydrogen ion concentration; practically, a scale of the acidity or alkalinity of substances. The neutral point is pH 7. Below 7, acidity increases. Above 7, alkalinity increases.
Phaeochromocytoma	A tumour, usually arising in the inner part of the adrenal gland, which secretes excessive amounts of hormones, producing such symptoms as tremor, cramps, palpatations, headache, nausea, and high blood pressure. Treatment is surgical removal.
Phalanx	One of the bones of the fingers or toes. The plural is *phalanges*.
Phantom limb	The illusion that a limb which has been amputated is still attached to the body and feels pain and other sensations.
Pharmacopoeia	An authoritative collection of formulas and methods of preparing and using drugs, which sets standards of purity, safety, and potency.
Pharyngeal tonsils	Lymphoid tissue better known as *adenoids*.
Pharyngitis	Sore throat.
Pharynx	The membrane-lined cavity at the back of the nose, mouth, and throat; the place where a sore throat hurts.
Phenylalanine	An essential AMINO ACID, present in protein foods.
Phenylketonuria	Hereditary inability to metabolize phenylalanine, an essential amino acid, because of a genetically determined lack of a neccessary enzyme; an inherited error of metabolism. Breakdown products of incompletely metabolized phenylalanine accumulate in the infant's body and impair brain function. The

Guthrie test of an infant's blood gives evidence of the condition soon after birth. A diet of special foods, very low in phenylalanine, lessens the threat of damage to the developing nervous system.

Tightness of the foreskin of the penis, preventing retraction over the tip of the organ.

Phimosis

Inflammation of the walls of a vein, which may lead to formation of a clot, *thrombophlebitis*.

Phlebitis

Formation of a clot in a vein. Not due to local inflammation.

Phlebothrombosis

Bloodletting, by cutting into a vein; venesection. Irrational bloodletting for almost any state of ill health was practised wholesale in the seventeenth and eighteenth centuries. The practice undoubtedly weakened and even caused the death of patients. It fell into deserved disrepute as a panacea. But there are some conditions for which bloodletting is recognized as a part of modern treatment; see HAEMOCHROMATOSIS and POLYCYTHAEMIA.

Phlebotomy

An abnormal, excessive dread or fear. There are scores of specific phobias, each with its own medical name.

Phobia

An instrument which measures the concentration of radioisotopes (measured doses of radiation) in a patient's body. See NUCLEAR MEDICINE.

Photoscanner

A number of disorders are caused or made worse by exposure to sunlight. Photosensitive reactions may result from certain drugs taken internally, from materials in cosmetics or substances applied to the skin, from contact with certain plants (parsnips, celery, carrots, dill, parsley), or from underlying disease which increases the sensitivity of the skin to sunlight. A clue to photosensitive reactions is the presence of lesions on exposed areas of the forehead, nose, edges of the ears, and backs of the hands, while areas under the jaw not exposed to sunlight are not affected. Patients with *lupus erythematosus*

Photosensitivity

are sensitive to sunlight.

Phototherapy	Treatment with light rays, including invisible ultraviolet and infrared wavelengths.
Phrenic nerve	The principal nerve of breathing which activates the muscle of respiration, the *diaphragm*. The nerve also serves the PERICARDIUM and PLEURA.
Phthisis	An old term for pulmonary tuberculosis.
Physical allergy	Allergic reactions induced by purely physical factors such as heat, cold, or light.
Phytobezoar	A compact ball of vegetable matter in the stomach.
Pia mater	The innermost of the three membranes that cover the brain and spinal cord.
Pica	A craving to eat strange foods or unnatural substances – wood, clay, coal, dirt, chalk, starch, and so on. Pica is more common in children.
Pigeon-breeder's lung	A recently recognized respiratory disease occurring in pigeon breeders or others in close contact with pigeons. Chills, fever, cough, and shortness of breath develop a few hours after inhaling dusts in an environment of pigeons. The disease is not a bacterial or viral infection, but appears to be a hypersensitivity reaction to ANTIGENS in pigeon feathers and droppings, a disease similar to FARMER'S LUNG.
Pigeon toe	Inward turning of the feet and toes when walking. Children in the early stages of walking are often pigeon-toed but usually outgrow the condition.
Piles	See HAEMORRHOIDS.
Pill rolling	Involuntary movement of thumb and finges, as if a pill were being rolled, a feature of Parkinson's disease.

A congenital hair-containing sac under the skin overlying the coccyx at the top of the cleft of the buttock. There may be only a dimpling of the skin or a hairy overlying tuft to mark the presence of the cyst until it becomes infected, swollen, and painful, and perhaps develops a FISTULA through which fluids are excreted. Surgical removal of the cyst is usually neccessary to accomplish a permanent cure.

Pilonidal cyst

The term for what doctors call a *pustule*.

Pimple

A structure about a quarter of an inch long which lies very nearly in the centre of the brain. For centuries physiologists were unable to ascribe any function to it. Now there is evidence that the pineal is a sort of biological clock which influences the activities of hormones. Experiments with animals indicate that in some way the pineal regulates the sex glands.

Pineal gland

One variety of acute *conjunctivitis*, a highly contagious infection of the eye. Discharges contain the infective organisms.

Pink eye

The external ear; the protruding part of the hearing mechanism, mainly a sound collector.

Pinna

Threadworms, oxyuriasis.

Pinworm infection

A noninfectious, noncontagious skin disease of young adults, characterized by scaly patches.

Pityriasis rosea

An inert substance such as a sugar pill, without drug effect, given to please the patient or as a comparison with a drug being tested. Oddly, seeming therapeutic benefits and even side effects from placebos are not uncommon. The phenomenon, called the placebo effect, has to be taken account of in the evaluation of drug effects.

Placebo

The organ on the wall of the uterus through which the fetus receives nourishment and eliminates wastes. Structures of the implanted embryo grow into the uterine wall and the placenta develops until it occupies about half the area of the uterus at the fourth month of pregnancy. The fetus and placenta are

Placenta

connected by the UMBILICAL CORD. The placenta has a definite life span and is a senile organ by the time labour pains begin. It is expelled as the AFTERBIRTH shortly after the baby is born. It is flat, about an inch thick and six or seven inches in diameter. Complications of pregnancy may be caused by a mislocated placenta (*placenta praevia*) or by premature detachment.

Plague	An acute feverish disease caused by bacilli (*Pasteurella pestis*). It is primarily a disease of rats and other rodents, which tend to be inhabited by fleas, which can transmit plague to man. *Bubonic plague* is characterized by swellings (*buboes*) under the arms and in the groins. *Pneumonic plague* affects the lungs and has a high fatality rate. The plague, or Black Death, which ravaged Europe in the fourteenth century, was a form of bubonic plague with an exceptionally high incidence of haemorrhage.
Plantar	Of or relating to the soles of the feet. The most frequent affliction of this area is *plantar warts* which usually form at points of pressure on the ball of the foot.
Plantar reflex (*Babinski sign*)	Upward movement of the big toe and downward movement of the other toes when the sole of the foot is stroked; an indication of certain nervous system disorders.
Plaque	Patches or unnatural formations on tissues such as on tooth surfaces and on inner arterial walls. *Atheroma*, plaques that are found in walls of arteries, contain some LIPIDS and some connective or scar tissue. They contribute to stiffening of blood vessel walls, narrowing of arteries, choking of circulation, and ruptured arteries, associated with heart attacks.
Plasma	The fluid part of the blood, minus the blood cells.
Plasma cell	A type of white blood cell closely related to *lymphocytes*. Multiple MYELOMA and a form of leukaemia are associated with plasma cell abnormalities.
Plasmodium	The genus of parasites that cause malaria, transmitted by the

bites of mosquitoes.

Tiny, colourless structures in the blood, about a quarter of the size of a red blood cell, which help to initiate blood clotting. They are formed in the bone marrow. Platelets are fragile and short-lived outside the circulation, and there are various methods of salvaging and transfusing them. *Platelet transfusions* may be necessary in some bleeding disorders such as *purpura*. Platelet transfusions may be of fresh whole blood, or of recently stored blood collected in specially treated glass containers or plastic bags. Since it is the platlets themselves rather than whole blood which the patient usually requires, a recently developed procedure promises to be less wasteful of hospital blood bank supplies. Platelets for transfusion are separated from blood given by a donor, and the donor's blood, minus the platelets, is returned to his circulation. The donor soon makes new platelets.	**Platelets** (*thrombocytes*)
The thin, glistening membrane attached to the outer surface of the lungs and the inner surface of the chest wall. The opposed fluid-lubricated surfaces glide over each other as the lung contracts and expands, so that breathing is painless.	**Pleura**
Inflammation of the pleura, causing knifelike pains aggravated by a deep breath or coughing. There are wet and dry forms of pleurisy.	**Pleurisy**
Sharp pain in the muscles between the ribs. It is characteristic of *Bornholm disease*, an acute virus-caused epidemic disease.	**Pleurodynia**
LEAD POISONING.	**Plumbism**
Chronic inflammation of the lungs, due to long-continued inhalation of various kinds of mineral dusts.	**Pneumoconiosis**
Removal of an entire lung.	**Pneumonectomy**
Inflammation of the lungs caused by various organisms. In the past it was customary to classify pneumonias according to the	**Pneumonia**

part of the lung affected – *lobar pneumonia* if a lobe or lobes were involved, *bronchopneumonia* if infection was localized to air sacs connecting with bronchi. Now the trend is to classify pneumonia according to the organism that causes it. A common causative organism is the pneumococcus. The terms *viral pneumonia* and *primary atypical pneumonia* came into vogue after World War II to describe pneumonias not caused by recognized bacteria. Viruses may be implicated, but it is now known that most cases of atypical pneumonia are caused by *mycoplasma*. These are strange organisms like bacteria, but they lack the stiff outer covering that holds conventional bacteria in shape and are enveloped only in a flexible membrane. During the progress of research the organisms have been called *Eaton's agent* and *pleuropneumonia-like organisms* (PPLO), the latter because they resemble organisms which cause a respiratory disease of cattle called pleuropneumonia. They have recently been given a category of their own, the genus *mycoplasma*. Respiratory infection caused by these germs comes on gradually, producing fever, chills, and cough. The patient does not appear to be very ill, and often does not consult a doctor, although he may stay at home from work for a few days with a 'bad cold." The organisms are sensitive to tetracycline, an antibiotic. Another form of *pneumonia*, of which the cause may not be immediately suspected, is parrot fever (*ornithosis, psittacosis*), an infection transmitted by parrots and other birds. Other unusual pneumonias may result from foreign material that gets into the lungs; see ASPIRATION PNEUMONIA.

Pneumothorax Collapse of a lung due to air in the pleural cavity.

Podagra Gout.

Poisonous plants Any plant that is not a familiar food plant is poisonous if parts of it are eaten. That is the safest rule to follow, even though parts of some strange or common plants may be harmless. Children are particularly attracted by berries which look good to eat but may be highly poisonous. They should be taught never to chew or eat unknown berries, leaves, roots, or barks. Many highly toxic plants are cultivated in gardens; others, some of them quite attractive, grow wild. A partial list of toxic plants includes many cultivated for their beauty: foxglove leaves and seeds, poinsettia leaves, oleander leaves and branches, iris roots, larkspur, delphinium, lily of the valley, monkshood, yew, daphne, Christmas rose, bittersweet. Bulbs of hyacinth, narcissus, and daffodil are toxic; as purchased, plant bulbs may be treated with toxic chemicals. Rhubarb leaves (the stalks are edible), wisteria seeds, any part of laurels, rhododendrons, and azaleas can produce serious poisoning. Play safe by never putting any part of a growing plant into the mouth. Immediate treatment of plant poisoning is emptying of the stomach by inducing vomiting, unless the victim is unconscious or having a fit, and calling a doctor.

Measurements of the number of pollen particles in the air at a given time, made by counting the numbers of particles adhering to a glass slide covered with sticky material and exposed to the atmosphere.	**Pollen counts**
A state of allergic reaction to inhaled plant pollens; for example, hay fever, asthma.	**Pollinosis**
A rare disease characterized by inflammation and nodular swellings of artery walls, sometimes leading to local death of tissues. Also called *periarteritis nodosa* and *polyarteritis nodosa*. The cause is not known.	**Polyarteritis**
A congenital developmental defect in which the kidneys are filled with bubble-like cysts.	**Polycystic kidney**
Too many red cells in the blood.	**polycythaemia**
More than the normal number of fingers or toes.	**Polydactyly**
Enormous thirst, characteristic of *diabetes insipidus*, and sometimes of *diabetes mellitus*.	**Polydipsia**
Smooth outgrowths or tumours of mucous membranes which line body cavities. Usually the polyp hangs from a stem or stalk. Polyps occur most commonly in mucous tissues of the	**Polyps**

nose, uterus, and colon. They rarely cause symptoms, but nasal polyps may be associated with allergies, and some polyps, as of the colon, may be precancerous and are best removed when discovered. Surgical removal is relatively simple.

Polyunsaturated fats

Much interest has been aroused by well-publicized knowledge that high levels of CHOLESTEROL in the blood may be reduced by increasing the proportion of polyunsaturated fats in the diet. The hope is that reduction of blood cholesterol may slow the process of *arteriosclerosis* which leads to heart attacks. It is not possible to speak with complete assurance about prevention of an extremely complex and incompletely understood process, but most authorities agree that it is unwise to flood the body with large amounts of unsaturated fats. Saturated is a technical word referring to bonds between the carbon atoms of fatty acids which combine with glycerol to form fats and oils. These bonds in *saturated fats* contain all the hydrogen atoms they can hold. *Unsaturated* and *polyunsaturated* fatty acids have additional bonds between carbon atoms and can take on additional atoms; thus they are more chemically active. Most of the animal fats and some of the vegetable oils (for example, coconut oil) are formed from fatty acids which are highly saturated. Fish oils, corn oil, sunflower oil, cottonseed oil, and some other vegetable oils are highly unsaturated. The polyunsaturated fatty acid of principal nutritional importance is *linoleic acid*. Most of the fat stored in the adult human body is relatively unsaturated.

Polyuria

Excessive output of urine.

Popliteal

Of or relating to the hind part of the knee joint.

Portuguese man-of-war

Creatures that people call jellyfish sometimes empty beaches in a hurry. The most formidable, not exactly a jellyfish, is the Portuguese man-of-war, a creature – actually composed of many separate organisms – which floats on the surface and drapes scores of tentacles into the depths. The tentacles, as long as 50 feet, contain venom-injecting surfaces for killing prey. The stingers feel like a hot iron to the bather who comes into contact with them. There is immediate pain, burning, feeling of tightness in the chest, and nausea after a minute or so. The muscles cramp and it feels as if every muscle of the body is contracting. The stung areas should be flushed with water while medical help is on the way. The skin may be rubbed with a cloth, or better still, lathered and shaved with a safety razor to remove venomous particles. Antihistamine drugs seem to give the most rapid relief of pain, cramping, and spasm. Persons with weak hearts may be dangerously affected by the man-of-war toxin and should have prompt medical care.

After childbirth.	**Postpartum**
After a meal. *Postcibal* has the same meaning.	**Postprandial**
Use of gravity to assist in draining secretions from the lungs and chest. The patient lies face down over the edge of a bed or table, his head, shoulders, and chest hanging down lower than the waist. In this position, gravity helps to drain secretions. Coughing, and thumping the back encourage drainage.	**Postural drainage**
Of or relating to the area of the chest overlying the heart. Precordial pain may or may not come from the heart; there are many structures in this area.	**Precordial**
Forerunner; something that precedes. In biology, a compound that can be used by the body to form another compound. For example, the body converts vegetable *carotene* into vitamin A.	**Precursor**
Cyclic occurrence of emotional symptoms associated with body changes about a week before onset of a menstrual period. Most women are aware of some change in disposition during the premenstrual week and learn to live with it, but some have sufficient distress to seek medical attention. Nervous symptoms such as irascibility, tension, fatigue, moodiness, weeping, severe enough to upset domestic tranquillity, are not all in the mind but reflect bodily changes. Physical symptoms such as abdominal swelling, weight gain, swelling of the hands, and	**Premenstrual tension**

swelling and tenderness of the breasts, indicate that the fundamental disturbance which provokes emotional irritability is cyclic OEDEMA – transitory retention of fluids, which exert pressure on internal organs and have far-reaching effects. The tension state ends at the onset of menstruation. A doctor may prescribe diuretics, sedatives, stimulants, or other measures according to individual need. Explanation that premenstrual tension is not abnormal is reassuring.

Prenatal	Before birth.
Prepuce	A fold of skin covering the head (glans) of the **penis** or CLITORIS; the foreskin; the part that is removed in circumcision.
Presbycusis	Normal diminution of acuteness of hearing that comes with increasing age. Mainly, sensitivity to the highest sound frequencies is reduced while sensitivity to lower frequencies – those most important in conversation and daily affairs – remains good.
Presbyopia	The change in eyesight caused by ageing. It begins to come on in middle life when the lens of the eye loses some of its elasticity and power of ACCOMMODATION. Near objects have to be held farther away to see them distinctly. In a culture that depends on reading, close vision, and paperwork, corrective glasses are a necessity and an aid to efficiency.
Pressure sores	Sores or ulcers resulting from pressure on parts of the body in persons confined to bed for long periods; good nursing care can do much to relieve and prevent them.
Priapism	Abnormal, painful, sustained erection of the PENIS, unrelated to sexual stimuli. It may result from obstruction of vessels that drain the organ, from injury to nerve centres, or from stimuli such as bladder stones or PROSTATITIS.
Prickly heat	See MILIARIA.
Primary irritants	Caustic, acid, corrosive, or otherwise irritating substances

which are harmful to anyone's skin on first exposure in sufficient concentration; no allergic reaction is involved.

Premonitory; early warning signs of an oncoming condition before overt symptoms appear.	**Prodromal**
A doctor's forecast of the course and duration of an illness based on the best information available to make a judgment.	**Prognosis**
Forceful ejection of stomach contents.	**Projectile vomiting**
A hormone of the pituitary gland which stimulates milk production.	**Prolactin**
A falling downward of a part from its normal position; for example, *prolapse of the uterus.*	**Prolapse**
Prevention of the spread or development of disease, for example by public health measures, vaccination, or inoculation against infections.	**Prophylaxis**
A group of hormone-like substances which occur in minute amounts in virtually all body tissues. The name, something of a misnomer, originated with discovery of the substances in semen, to which the prostate gland contributes. Different prostaglandins (at least sixteen natural forms are known) have different and even opposite effects. Prostaglandins are so versatile that many investigators expect them to become major therapeutic agents if experimental and clinical trials prove their safety and effectiveness in a wide range of conditions. Prostaglandins stimulate or relax smooth muscle, appear to regulate cell behaviour, and inhibit and potentiate hormones. On the evidence of clinical and experimental studies, specific prostaglandins may become valuable drugs for: induction of labour at term; contraception; induced abortion; prevention and treatment of peptic ulcer (by shutting off gastric secretions); induction of delayed menstruation; control of high blood pressure; treatment of bronchial asthma, emphysema, even the common cold (by opening closed airways). Aspirin	**Prostaglandins**

tends to halt production of prostaglandins, which sheds some light on the way aspirin works. Various prostaglandins can cause fever, inflammation, and headache, symptoms commonly relieved by aspirin.

Prostatectomy	Removal of all or part of the *prostate gland* by surgical operation.
Prostatitis	Acute or chronic inflammation of the *prostate gland*.
Prosthesis	A substitute for a missing part of the body; for example, artificial eye, limb, or denture.
Prosthodontics	The branch of dentistry that relates to the replacement of missing teeth and oral structures by artificial devices.
Proteins	Large complex molecules built up of long chains of simpler AMINO ACIDS. Skin, hair, nails, muscles are largely protein. It is the characteristic matter of life. Enzymes which carry out multitudes of living chemical processes of the body are proteins. About one half of the dry weight of the body is protein. Protein constituents of foods are broken down into their constituent amino acids by digestion, assimilated, and the separated parts are reassembled by body cells into specific and unique personal proteins (SEE GENES, HEREDITY). Bodily synthesis of proteins is essential not only for growth and repair of tissues but for the continuance of the multitudes of chemical processes we live by. Protein elements of foods can be burned for energy if necessary, but carbohydrates and fats are superior energy providers.
Prothrombin	A plasma PROTEIN, one of many elements necessary in the complicated processes of blood coagulation. Tests of prothrombin time are used in patients having a tendency to haemorrhage and as a guide to treatment of patients receiving anticoagulant drugs.
Protoplasm	Living matter; the material which is the essential matter of living cells, never found in the inanimate world. The word was meaningful years ago when the best that scientists could do

was to analyse the cell constituents – carbohydrates, proteins, fats, salts, water, and so on – of what they considered to be one substance. Today, many of the structures and activities of specific elements of protoplasm are known – mechanisms of heredity, protein synthesis, energy transformations, chemical directives of life – and the word is outliving its usefulness except as a very general term for living matter.

Single-celled organisms. Most protozoa do not cause disease, but those that do are responsible for malaria, amoebic dysentery, and a number of other diseases.	**Protozoa**
Plastic surgery to correct protruding, flattened, or deformed ears is usually performed on children, but is just as suitable for adults. The operation (*otoplasty*) is performed by means of incisions behind the ears. The procedure takes from an hour to an hour and a half. The patient may be discharged from the hospital as soon as 24 hours after surgery. A bandage is worn over the ears for about one week after surgery, and the ear is further protected during sleeping for another two weeks.	**Protruding ears**
An excess of GRANULATION TISSUE.	**Proud flesh**
A chronic skin ailment characterized by small, deep-seated, solid pimples that itch intensely.	**Prurigo**
Severe itching.	**Pruritus**
A hallucinogenic drug.	**Psilocybin**
A pneumonia-like disease transmitted by infected birds. The disease affects not only birds of the parrot family, but pigeons, chickens, ducks, turkeys, and other birds.	**Psittacosis** (*ornithosis, parrot fever*)
A chronic disease of the skin, of unknown cause, usually persisting for years with periods of remission and recurrence. It is characterized by elevated lesions in various parts of the body – elbows, knees, scalp, nails, lower back – covered with dry silvery scales that drop off. General health is rarely affected, although *psoriatic arthritis*, a form of arthritis in the	**Psoriasis**

fingers and toes, may develop in some patients.

Psychedelic	The word means mind-manifesting, and is applied to drugs which affect the mood and the mind.
Psychoanalysis	A system of mental therapy created by Sigmund Freud, originally as a research method to gain insight into mental processes. Essentially, the patient speaks to the psychoanalyst about whatever comes in mind, during a long series of sessions which usually total several hundred hours for a complete analysis. Unconscious conflicts expressed through dreams, slips of the tongue, symbolism, and so on, are interpreted by the psychoanalyst with the object of giving the patient insight into his conflicts and thus lessening their injurious effects. The therapeutic value of psycholanalysis is controversial.
Psychomotor seizure	A relatively mild form of epileptic attack which the patient never remembers. He does not fall but may stagger, make restless movements and strange sounds, and lose contact with his environment for a minute or two.
Psychoneurosis	An emotionally based disturbance of the personality, often severe enough to be handicapping, generally a defensive reaction to psychological conflicts.
Psychosis	Serious mental illness, disabling, usually requiring treatment in a hospital. Some psychoses have organic causes and others primarily psychological causes or possibly metabolic disturbances too subtle to be identifiable.
Psychosomatic disease	A disease, sometimes but not always without accompanying physical causes, in which disturbing emotions of the patient play an important part in inciting, worsening, or continuing the disability.
Psychosurgery	Operations on parts of the brain to alter a personality. *Prefrontal lobotomy,* an operation in which the frontal lobes of the brain are cut into, at one time had many advocates. Unmanageable, violent, manic patients subjected to this procedure usually become tractable and even amiable, but too often with

gross deterioration of personality to a vegetative level. Psycho-surgery is a drastic procedure that is resorted to only when other measures have failed.

Treatment of emotional and mental disorders by psychological methods as opposed to physical or medical methods.	**Psychotherapy**
Putrid substances produced by decay of dead animal matter. Food poisoning is not caused by ptomaines, which are too malodorous for anyone to digest. Food poisoning is commonly caused by salmonella or staphylococcus organisms.	**Ptomaines**
An enzyme in saliva which initiates the digestion of starch. *Ptyalism* is the condition of excess of saliva; salivation.	**Ptyalin**
The age at which the reproductive organs become functionally active. It occurs when a person is between twelve and seventeen years old and is indicated in the girl by the beginning of menstruation and in the boy by development of semen and deepening of the voice.	**Puberty**
The external sex organs.	**Pudenda**
The time of childbirth and return of the uterus to its pre-pregnancy size.	**Puerperium**
A disorder of blood coagulation; tiny blood vessels bleed into the skin and mucous membranes, and cause purplish patches to pinpoint haemorrhages. There are many causes.	**Purpura**
Containing, exuding, or producing pus.	**Purulent**
A fluid derived from the blood, containing many white cells, the response to certain infections.	**Pus**
A small elevation of the skin containing pus.	**Pustule**
Pus in the blood.	**Pyaemia**
An X-ray film showing the pelvis of the kidney and ureter.	**Pyelogram**

Pyelonephritis	Infection of the kidney and its urine-collecting pelvis.
Pyloric stenosis	In babies, obstruction of the outlet of the stomach due to abnormal thickening of the pyloric muscle that encircles it. The condition is completely relieved by an operation which cuts some of the muscle fibres. In adults, it usually arises from scarring or a growth.
Pylorospasm	Spasm of the circular muscle at the outlet of the stomach, manifested by PROJECTILE VOMITING of an infant shortly after birth. Usually the condition can be corrected by medication which relaxes the muscle and permits normal passage of food to the intestines.
Pyogenic	Pus-producing.
Pyorrhoea	Literally, flow of pus; a common term for *periodontoclasia*, inflammation and gradual destruction of supporting tissues of the teeth. Pockets form and enlarge between the gum surface and tooth, bacteria and debris fill the pockets, pus forms, and bone is absorbed. Eventually the tooth becomes loose in its socket and is lost from lack of support. The condition can be arrested but lost tissue cannot be restored.
Pyrexia	Fever.
Pyridoxine	One of the B vitamins, commonly designated as vitamin B_6.
Pyrosis	Heartburn.
Pyuria	Pus in the urine.

Q

A self-limiting disease caused by RICKETTSIAE, resembling pneumonia, often mild and unrecognized.	**Q fever**
Four times a day.	**Q.i.d.**
The large muscle which extends the thigh.	**Quadriceps**
Paralysis of both arms and both legs.	**Quadriplegia**
A tender, vital part, such as the bed of a fingernail.	**Quick**
The time about the middle of pregnancy when kicks and flutters within the uterus give unmistakable evidence that life is present.	**Quickening**
An abscess in and around a tonsil, causing a very sore throat.	**Quinsy**
Occurring every day – usually referring to fever.	**Quotidian**

A lethal disease caused by viruses which have an affinity for brain and nervous tissue. The virus is transmitted to man by the bite of an infected (rabid) animal. Mere contact of an infected animal with abraded or scratched skin can transmit the disease. Mad dogs are not the only sources of rabies. A considerable reservoir exists in wildlife in certain areas. Bats, foxes, squirrels, and other rabid animals can transmit the disease directly by biting people or indirectly by infecting domestic animals which in turn can transmit the disease by their bites or saliva. The disease is invariably fatal but has an incubation period of a month to a year or more. The incubation period is shortest if bites are inflicted on the head, face, neck, or arms, and are severe and numerous. Prompt Pasteur treatment – daily injection of rabies vaccine for two weeks – usually prevents rabies from taking hold. The treatments are painful and the type of vaccine cultivated in animal nerve tissue sometimes has bad side affects. A newer type of duck-embryo rabies vaccine greatly reduces the serious problem of nervous system reactions. Immediate preventive injections may not be necessary if the biting animal can be caught and kept under observation. If killed, the animal's body and particularly the head should be kept for laboratory studies which can determine whether or not the animal was rabid. If injections have been started, and the animal proves not to be rabid, they can be discontinued. The problem of what to do about the bite of a possibly rabid animal should be turned over immediately to the doctor and local health department.

Rabies (*hydrophobia*)

Illness resulting from intense or cumulative exposure to sources of radiation. Exposure to massive doses of radiation, as in the neighbourhood of a nuclear explosion, is very rare. An overwhelming dose of radiation is extremely serious if not fatal. Necessary therapeutic use of X-rays may sometimes be followed by mild radiation sickness – lassitude, nausea, vomiting – which usually disappears quickly and can be coped with effectively by the physician or radiologist. There is virtually no threat of radiation sickness from the use of diagnostic X-rays.

Radiation sickness

Inflammation of a spinal nerve root.

Radiculitis

Radiograph	An X-ray photograph.
Radioisotopes	See NUCLEAR MEDICINE.
Radiologist	A physician who specializes in the making and interpretation of X-ray studies and applications of radiation.
Radiopaque	Not transparent to X-rays. Radiopaque substances (for example, BARIUM MEAL) are introduced into parts of the body to give clear delineation of structures which otherwise would not show up distinctly on an X-ray film or fluoroscopic screen.
Radiosensitivity	The capacity of tissues to react with different degrees of intensity to radiation. This quality is used in the treatment of some kinds of cancer.
Radiotherapy	Treatment of disease by X-rays, radium, radioisotopes, and other forms of ionizing radiation.
Radon	A radioactive gas given off by the decay of radium. *Radon* seeds are tiny radon-containing tubes of gold or glass for implantation into tumours. The gas decays at a steady rate and after a week or so loses all its radioactive power, so no harm is done if radon seeds remain in or are lost in tissues.
Rales	Abnormal sounds from the lungs or air passageways, heard over the chest. The sounds, described as coarse, medium, fine, wet, dry, and so on, are not specific but help the doctor to judge the condition of the patient.
Raynaud's disease	Intermittent blanching and reddening of the skin, especially of the fingers, brought on by exposure to cold. Blood vessels first constrict, causing pallor and numbness, the affected area becomes blue and then red as large amounts of blood return. An attack may last for minutes or hours. The condition may be secondary to other diseases, but more often the peculiar blood vessel spasms occur without apparent cause; 90 per cent of patients are women. There is some evidence that affected persons may be unusually susceptible to collagen diseases such

as SCLERODERMA in later life, but in itself Raynaud's disease is more a nuisance than a serious condition. Patients are usually instructed to protect themselves well against cold, by wearing warm clothes, lined gloves, and overshoes, because a certain amount of exposure to cold is necessary to trigger attacks. Smoking which tends to constrict superficial vessels, is forbidden. In its most extreme form, Raynaud's disease may lead to dry GANGRENE of the fingers. Surgical severing of nerves which serve blood vessels of affected areas may be resorted to in patients with severe symptoms.

A bulging of the rectum through the rear wall of the vagina.	**Rectocele**
The terminal part of the bowel, about six inches long, ending in the narrow muscular anal canal and anus.	**Rectum**
The palms often become deep pink or reddish, like a sustained blush, during pregnancy. The reddening, caused by a high level of circulating hormones, fades after delivery and needs no treatment. A similar phenomenon occurs in some patients with cirrhosis of the liver.	**Red palms** (palmar erythema)
A type of cell characteristic of HODGKIN'S DISEASE.	**Reed-Sternberg cell**
Pain that does not originate where it hurts. For instance, pain which originates in an inflamed gallbladder may be felt in the back under the right shoulder blade.	**Referred pain**
An action in response to a stimulus, occurring without conscious effort or thinking about it; for example, dilatation or contraction of the pupil in response to different intensities of light. Some 300 different reflexes have been catalogued. They are useful in helping to diganose or locate the sites of disorders, infections, or injuries that may involve the nervous system.	**Reflex**
Bending of light waves from a straight line in passing through lenses or transparent structures of different densities. In ophthalmology, the measurement and correction by lenses of defects of the eye (*shortsightedness, longsightedness, astigma-*	**Refraction**

tism) which prevents light waves from being brought to a sharp focus exactly on the retina.

Regional ileitis
(*Crohn's disease*)

Inflammatory disease of the lower portion of the small bowel. The disease may be principally inflammatory, obstructive, or diffuse, with varied symptoms. Total recovery may be made after a single attack and there may be no symptoms for many years although abnormalities of the small bowel still persist. Medical treatment usually is effective but complications may require surgery.

Regurgitation

Effortless bringing up of food from the stomach soon after eating; spitting up of food. Babies are adept at it. Not to be mistaken for vomiting. The word also means backflow of blood through a leaky heart valve.

Reiter's syndrome

A form of arthritis with inflammation of the mucous membrane of the eyes and of the urethra. It resembles rheumatoid arthritis but in many respects is less crippling and is self-limiting.

Relapsing fever

Episodes of fever which subside spontaneously, then recur. Specifically, an acute infectious disease caused by organisms spread by lice and ticks.

Renal insufficiency

Incapacity of the kidneys to filter toxins adequately from the blood.

Renin

A kidney protein capable of raising blood pressure by activating *angiotensin*, a powerful pressure-elevating agent.

Resect

To cut out a part of an organ or tissue; a term used by surgeons.

Residual urine

Significant amount of urine left in the bladder after urination. This symptom in men may be associated with prostate trouble; in women, with CYSTOCELE or pressure of tumours of the uterus.

Respirator

A mechanical breathing device for patients whose breathing

muscles are paralysed by disease or injury.

See HYALINE MEMBRANE DISEASE.	**Respiratory distress syndrome**

Artificial respiration applied to a person suffering from asphyxia. **Resuscitation**

A pervasive mechanism like a network throughout the body, which defends against foreign invaders. **Reticuloendothelial system**

The fine light-receiving structure at the back of the eye, composed of ten layers. Hundreds of thousands of nerve endings in the retina merge into the optic nerve which conveys impulses to the seeing part of the brain at the back of the head. **Retina**

Hereditary degeneration and atrophy of the retina. **Retinitis pigmentosa**

A malignant tumour of the retina; a congenital form of cancer occurring in infants and young children. An early sign is a white pupil; this sign in an infant or young child has serious import and immediate medical diagnosis is imperative. Retinoblastoma is life-threatening, but improved methods of treatment, given as soon as the tumour is discovered, usually save life though sometimes at the cost of partial or total blindness. If only one eye is affected, it is usually removed. If both eyes are involved the more seriously affected one is usually removed and the other is treated in the hope of destroying the tumour and preserving as much vision as possible. X-rays, radioactive applicators, photocoagulation, and other measures may be used in an effort to save the eye. The disease is thought to be inherited as a dominant trait. **Retinoblastoma**

Any abnormal condition of the retina. **Retinopathy**

Instruments designed to hold or pull back the edges of an incision or wound. **Retractors**

Behind the eyeball. **Retrobulbar**

Retroflexion	Condition of being bent backwards.
Retroversion	A backward-tilted position of an organ, as a retroverted uterus.
Rh disease	See ERYTHROBLASTOSIS.
Rheumatism	A general term for painful, disabling conditions affecting the joints, muscles, and surrounding structures.
Rheumatoid factor	An abnormal PROTEIN in the blood of about 70 per cent of patients with *rheumatoid arthritis*. The rheumatoid factor acts like an ANTIBODY against one of the patient's own normal body proteins, with resulting inflammation and damage to tissue. This is much like an acquired allergy to a part of one's self. Mechanism which produce the rheumatoid factor have not been proved to be a cause of rheumatoid arthritis, but better knowledge about the factor may throw light on the fundamental nature of the disease. Tests for the factor are commonly given in diagnosing a suspected case of rheumatoid arthritis.
Rhinitis	Inflammation of the mucous membranes of the nose. It may arise from something as common as a cold, or from infections or allergies.
Rhinophyma	Overgrowth of blood vessels, sebaceous glands, connective tissue, and skin of the nose, giving the enlarged organ a knobbly, reddish, bulbous appearance. The condition is sometimes associated with overindulgence in spirits. Correction is surgical.
Rhinoplasty	Plastic surgery of the nose, for cosmetic purposes or correction of deformities.
Rhinorrhoea	Running nose.
Rhinoviruses	A family of 30 or more viruses which are major causes of the common cold.

R

A purple pigment in the retina. It is bleached on exposure to light and requires vitamin A for regeneration.

Rhodopsin

A method of contraception which relies on abstinence from sexual intercourse during the fertile phase of the menstrual cycle. OVULATION OCCURS around the midpoint of the menstrual cycle; the fertile period of about one week is assumed to span this midpoint, during which abstinence is practiced. If the menstrual cycle is regularly 28 days in length, the fertile period can be counted as beginning eleven days after onset of menstruation and continuing through the eighteenth day (or for extra assurance, beginning on day ten and continuing to day twenty). Menstrual cycles are rarely of exactly the same duration month after month. Calendar records may give a reasonably good average over several months, but if swings are great the accuracy of calculations is lessened. Some subjective signs suggest, but do not positively prove, that an egg has been released and that conception is possible; see OVULATION. In general, for couples who adopt the rhythm method, the safest period when conception is unlikely is the few days just before and just after menstruation.

Rhythm method
(calendar method)

A diet providing about ten ounces of boiled rice a day, with fruit juices and sugar, introduced in 1949 as an adjunct to the treatment of patients with severe high blood pressure. Benefits of the diet have been attributed largely to its very low sodium (salt) content. Since the introduction of antihypertensive and diuretic drugs, it is usually no longer necessary to restrict salt intake drastically.

Rice diet

A vitamin DEFICIENCY DISEASE of infants, resulting from insufficient dietary vitamin D or insufficient exposure to sunshine, which creates vitamin D from substances in the skin. Infantile rickets is manifested by distortion, softening, and bending of incompletely mineralized bones and sometimes by nodules strung like beads over the ribs. *Renal rickets* is not a deficiency disease but a congenital incapacity of the kidneys to reabsorb the phosphate necessary for normal bone structure.

Rickets

Disease-causing microbes smaller than bacteria but larger than

Rickettsiae

viruses. They are transmitted to man by the bites of fleas, ticks, and lice. Among the diseases they cause are *typhus*, *trench fever*, and *Q fever*.

Rifampicin

A recent addition to the antituberculosis drugs; a synthetic antibiotic which, in combination with at least one other well-known drug (*isoniazid, streptomycin, ethambutol*) is effective in eliminating tubercle bacilli from the sputum of most patients in about twenty weeks.

Ringworm

Infection by various fungi of the skin, hair, nails, and scalp. The troubles they cause have a general medical name, *dermatophytosis*, and a general word, tinea, linked with a name for the affected area, as *tinea capitis, tinea barbae, tinea pedis* (the last is better known as athlete's foot).

Rodent ulcer

A form of skin cancer (*basal cell epithelioma*), which does not spread to other areas of the body but which, if long neglected, tends to penetrate deeply and erode soft tissues and bones. The ulcers occur on sun-exposed areas of the face, especially at margins of the eyes, lips, nose, and ears. The edges of the ulcer have a rolled appearance. The lesion usually begins as a single pinhead to pea-sized nodule, waxy or pearly, which slowly enlarges by development of other waxy nodules near it and coalesce with them. In early stages before undermining of skin and bones begins, surgical removal or X-ray treatment is effective and leaves little scarring.

Roentgen

A quantitative unit of X-radiation, used in measuring intensity of exposure.

Root canal

A small channel in the root of a tooth, continuous with the pulp chamber above it. A tooth dead or dying from injury to its pulp may sometimes be saved by root filling or root resection.

Rosacea

See ACNE ROSACEA

Roseola

Any rose-coloured eruption of the skin. *Roseola infantum* is a viral infection of young children producing a fever which lasts three or four days, after which the temperature falls to normal, a skin rash appears, and the child is well.

Indigestible food residues in the intestinal tract, mostly composed of cellulose. A reasonable amount of bulky material is a mechanical aid to intestinal function.

Roughage

Several varieties of worms that invade the human body, gaining entrance by their eggs or larvae in contaminated soil or by hand-to-mouth transmission. The largest of the species is *Ascaris lumbricoides*; roundworms of lesser size are HOOK- WORMS, WHIPWORMS, THREADWORMS. Good hygiene and cooking are preventative measures.

Roundworms

A substance from the salivary glands of bees, fed by the worker bees to the queen bee. No important nutrient has been reported to be present in royal jelly that cannot be obtained readily from ordinary foods. It has no therapeutic value.

Royal jelly

Any agent that makes the skin red.

Rubefacient

---

see GERMAN MEASLES.

Rubella

Measles.

Rubeola

A test of female fertility; also called *tubal insufflation*. It determines whether the FALLOPIAN TUBES through which egg cells are transported to the uterus are open or obstructed. A gas, usually carbon dioxide, is introduced through the cervix under pressure. An instrument records significant changes in pressure as the gas flows through. If the fallopian tubes are open, bubbles of gas pass into the abdominal cavity.

Rubin test

Wrinkles, folds, elevations, ridges of tissue, as of the linings of the stomach and vagina.

Rugae

Chronic discharge from an ear, a warning that serious infection may erupt at any time.

Running ear

See HERNIA

Rupture

Ruptured disc Protrusion of the pulpy, cushioning pad between vertebrae through a tear in the surrounding ligament.

S

Oral poliovirus vaccine for immunization against polio. It contains weakened live polio viruses which produce an inapparent infection that establishes long-lasting immunity.	**Sabin vaccine**
A pouch or baglike covering of an organ or tissue; for example, the pericardial sac of the heart, the sac of a cyst; hernia, or tumour.	**Sac**
Sac-shaped.	**Saccular**
Backache in the region of the sacroiliac joints. The sciatic nerve traverses this area and ligaments and muscles are subject to injury. Many mechanisms can produce low back pain; treatment depends upon determination of the cause.	**Sacroiliac strain**
A large triangular, curved bone of the lower back, just above the coccyx, composed of live vertebrae fused together. The sacrum forms the back wall of the bony pelvis. On each side of the sacrum is the hipbone, the *ilium*, and their junction with the sacrum forms the *sacroiliac joint*.	**Sacrum**
The days during the menstrual cycle when conception is not likely to occur. See RHYTHM METHOD.	**Safe period**
Erysipelas.	**St. Anthony's fire**
See CHOREA.	**St. Vitus' dance**
A condition produced by overdosage with drugs of the aspirin family (salicylates), causing ringing in the ears, rapid breathing, nausea, visual disturbances, dizziness.	**Salicylism**
The three saliva-producing glands on each side of the face; the *parotid* gland in front of and below the ear (the one that is affected in mumps); the *sublingual* gland under the tongue; and the nearby *submaxillary* or *submandibular* gland.	**Salivary glands**
Excessive secretion of saliva. Ordinary MOTION SICKNESS, irritation of the nervous system, poisoning, local inflammations, certain infectious diseases, and disturbances of the stomach or	**Salivation**

liver can produce it.

Salk vaccine

A killed-virus vaccine for establishing immunity to polio. It is given in spaced injections; booster doses are recommended every two years. Oral polio vaccine (see SABIN VACCINE) is considered to have superiority.

Salmonella

A family of bacteria which cause gastrointestinal infections. They are the most common causes of FOOD POISONING. There are some 400 varieties of salmonella, one of which produces typhoid fever. Most cases of salmonella food poisoning are not definitely identified. The most frequent symptom is gastroenteritis, ranging from a few cramps to fulminating diarrhoea. A small percentage of recovered patients become carriers of the infection. The organisms are widely distributed in eggs, poultry, and other products. Thorough heating, above 74°C (165°F) destroys the organisms.

Salpingitis

Inflammation of one or both FALLOPIAN TUBES (*oviducts*). Symptoms are pain in the lower abdomen, tenderness, discharge from the cervix.

Saphenous veins

Two large veins of the leg near the skin surface which sometimes become varicose.

Sarcoidosis

A disease of unknown cause, somewhat resembling tuberculosis. Small tumours arise in almost any tissue, but particularly in the lungs, skin, bones, eyes, lymphatic system, liver, and muscle. The nodules may persist more or less unchanged for years or they may heal and recur. Symptoms vary with the organs affected. There is no specific treatment, but steroids help.

Sarcoma

A form of cancer arising mainly from connective tissue. *Osteogenic* sarcoma is a bone tumour, usually requiring amputation of the part. *Ewing's* sarcoma of children and young adults affects the shafts of long bones; the outlook is poor. A somewhat similar tumour, *reticulum cell* sarcoma, is sensitive to X-rays, and treatment by irradiation or amputation offers a good chance of survival.

See POLYUNSATURATED FATS.	**Saturated fat**
Excessive sexual desire in the male.	**Satyriasis**
The itch; infestation with female mites that burrow tiny tunnels in the skin and lay eggs in them.	**Scabies**
A small boat-shaped bone of the wrist and of the ankle.	**Scaphoid**
The shoulder blade.	**Scapula**
Wedge-shaped deformation of parts of certain vertebrae; a relatively common cause of backache in adolescents.	**Scheuermann's disease**
A parasitic disease of the tropics acquired by wading in fresh water where free-swimming forms of a blood fluke penetrate the skin and migrate to various organs by the bloodstream. Snails, in which eggs of the parasite develop into free-swimming larvae, are reservoirs of the disease.	**Schistosomiasis** (*bilharzia*)
A small channel at the junction of the white of the eye and the cornea through which fluids drain from the chamber of the eye in front of the lens. Narrowing or blocking of the drainage channel builds up pressures within the eye (*glaucoma*). Damage caused by glaucoma cannot be repaired. Glaucoma may be kept from progressing by eye drops, or surgery may be necessary to reopen channels.	**Schlemm, canal of**
Not a disease, but a symptom: pain in the back of the thigh and leg along the course of the sciatic nerve. Sciatica may be a form of neuritis or severe forms may result from disc trouble.	**Sciatica**
Hard.	**Scirrhous**
The strong, elastic outer coat of the eye, visible in front as the white of the eye.	**Sclera**
A connective tissue disease of unknown cause. The first signs usually appear in the skin of the hands and feet, in patchy areas which gradually involve more and more of the body. The skin	**Scleroderma**

slowly becomes hard, thickened, stiff, smooth, and shiny. The face may become mask-like because of loss of flexibility. Internal organs – lungs, heart, digestive tract, kidneys – are progressively affected. There is no specific treatment.

Sclerosing agents

Substances injected to harden and close up blood vessels, as in varicose veins and haemorrhoids.

Sclerosis

Hardening of tissue, especially by overgrowth of fibrous tissue. The sclerosing process affects many kinds of tissues; for example, nerve tissue (*multiple sclerosis*) and linings of the arteries (*arteriosclerosis*). What initiates and perpetuates the process is not understood.

Scoliosis

Sideways curvature of the spine.

Scorbutus

SCURVY.

Scotoma

A blind or partially blind area in the field of vision, indicating some change in the optic nerve or retina requiring examination by an ophthalmologist. *Scintillating scotomas*, frequently coloured, which have saw-toothed shimmering edges and spread out from a small spot to a large area then disappear in a few minutes, are often migraine-like phenomena.

Scratch test

A skin test for allergic sensitivity, especially to inhaled and contacted substances, done by scratching test material lightly into the skin without drawing blood. If the patient is sensitive to the substance, a positive reaction appears within a few minutes.

Scrofula

Tuberculosis of lymph nodes of the neck. The affliction was once common but has almost vanished since the advent of modern methods of treating tuberculosis.

Scrotum

The pouch containing the testicles.

Scrub typhus

A feverish disease from eastern Asia, transmitted by mites.

Scurf

Minute skin particles shed by animals. Inhalation of scurf is a frequent cause of allergic reactions.

A DEFICIENCY DISEASE due to lack of vitamin C, easily preventable and curable by taking the vitamin. Advanced scurvy with its classic symptoms of spongy, bleeding gums, loose teeth, and haemorrhages under the skin is now rare, but mild scurvy due to monotonous diets, food aversion, or inadequate supplementation of infant foods is still encountered occasionally.	**Scurvy**
See MOTION SICKNESS.	**Seasickness**
A wen; a localized skin swelling produced by obstruction of the outlet of an oil-secreting gland.	**Sebaceous cyst**
Glands of the skin which secrete *sebum* or skin oil; usually associated with hair follicles. Their function is to waterproof the skin.	**Sebaceous glands**
Overproduction or change in quality of skin oil secreted by sebaceous glands, producing oily skin, crusts, or scales.	**Seborrhoea**
The rate at which red blood cells settle out of a prepared specimen of blood under laboratory conditions; useful in diagnosis of certain diseases.	**Sedimentation rate**
A disease that comes to an end all by itself in a limited time, such as an uncomplicated cold.	**Self-limiting**
The whitish secretion containing SPERMATOZOA which is ejaculated by the male during orgasm. It is a mixture of secretions of the testes and prostate gland, which contributes most of its bulk.	**Semen**
Three interconnecting fluid-filled canals of the inner ear which lie in planes at right angles to each other. Our sense of balance is located here. Fluid in the canals responds to movement and sends information over nerve pathways to the brain.	**Semicircular canals**
Shaped like a half moon, as the *semilunar valves* of the heart.	**Semilunar**

Seminal vesicles	Accessory part of the male reproductive system. The two pouchlike vesicles lie behind the bladder. Each consists of a single tube coiled upon itself. The vesicles store spermatozoa and secrete a fluid which is added to secretions of the testes. Infection of the vesicles is rare.
Seminoma	A tumour of the testicle.
S.E.N.	State-enrolled nurse.
Septal defects	Abnormal openings between chambers of the heart which permit blood to leak from one side of the heart to the other.
Septicaemia	Blood poisoning; fever, prostration, the reaction to growing bacteria in the blood. Since the advent of antibiotics, septicaemia is less common and more controllable.
Septum	A partition or wall between two compartments or cavities; for instance, the nasal septum which divides the nostrils.
Sequestrum	A small piece of dead bone which has become detached from its normal position.
Serum	The amber-coloured fluid of blood that remains after the blood has coagulated and the clot has shrunk. It contains ANTIBODIES to bacteria and toxins. This is the basis of serums and antitoxins for treatment of disease. Animals, commonly horses, are inoculated with gradually increasing doses of bacteria or toxins until they build up large amounts of corresponding antibodies. The animal's serum is withdrawn, purified, and injected to increase the person's resistance to a particular disease.
Serum sickness	A reaction to injected animal sera. The most common symptom is nettle rash. Some patients have a skin rash; some have fever, pain in the joints, enlarged lymph nodes. Serum sickness is closely related to ANAPHYLAXIS, but much milder, and symptoms do not appear until several days after contact with the offending serum.

Broad-based; as in a tumour that does not have a stem or stalk.	**Sessile**

Although sex is almost always evident at birth, there are borderline cases where anomalies of development make the true sex difficult to determine (see HERMAPHRODITE). A guide to determination of genetic sex has been found to be the presence or absence in the subject's body cells of minute particles called *chromatin bodies*, which are visible under a microscope. Female cells contain chromatin bodies. Male cells do not, although the chromatin may be undetectable rather than absent. The sex chromatin method has been used to predict the sex of an infant before birth by study of cells obtained from the fluid which surrounds the fetus.

Sex determination

Certain traits such as COLOUR BLINDNESS and HAEMOPHILIA show a form of inheritance called *sex-linkage*. For example, mothers who do not exhibit a trait may transmit it to their sons, who do exhibit it, but not to their daughters. However, the daughters may carry the trait, which is in turn manifested in their sons. There are many technical and complex differences in sex-linked transmission lines, but the general principle is fairly simple: sex-linked traits occur because the GENES for expressing them are located in the pair of sex CHROMOSOMES which all normal persons possess. A female has two X chromosomes, one from her mother and one from her father, in her pair (XX). A male has an X chromosome from his mother and a Y chromosome from his father (XY). The Y chromosome is smaller and contains fewer genes. Many genes in the X chromosome have no counterpart in the Y. If there is a defective gene in one X chromosome of a woman, she has another X which is likely to be normal and to suppress the defective gene trait (although she still carries it). But the same defective gene in a man's X chromosome is paired with a Y which has no complementary gene to neutralize the trait, which therefore is fully expressed.

Sex-linked heredity

See PANHYPOPITUITARISM.	**Sheehan's disease**
See BACILLARY DYSENTERY.	**Shigellosis**

Shingles (*herpes zoster*)

A virus infection of nerve endings, manifested in the skin by crops of small blisters. The face and trunk are most often affected. Red patches appear and develop into fluid-filled blisters which become dry and scabbed in four or five days and eventually heal. The skin should be kept clean and dry and a doctor can prescribe measures to relieve distress. Infection of one nerve may reach the eye and threaten to leave scars on the *cornea*; competent care is important. In older people, shingles is sometimes followed by painful long-lasting *neuralgia* that is difficult to treat. Viruses that cause shingles and chickenpox are thought to be identical. Some adults exposed to chickenpox have developed shingles.

Shoe dermatitis

Not all cases of dermatitis of the feet are due to athlete's foot. Some, which may be mistaken for common fungus infection of the feet, are instances of shoe dermatitis – sensitization and reaction to rubber, leather, dyes, adhesives, and innumerable substances used in the manufacture of shoes. The skin may be dry and scaly, or red and itchy, and crops of small blisters may develop. Sweating and maceration of the skin promote sensitization by irritant substances from the shoes. Shoe dermatitis may first be suspected when treatments for supposed athlete's foot do not give any benefit. Unlike fungus infection of the feet, shoe dermatitis does not affect the webs of the toes or cause crumbling of the nails. Shoe dermatitis may be suspected if both feet are affected in the same symmetrical pattern, which may correspond with the design of the shoes. If the irritation subsides when a particular pair of shoes is not worn, and flares up when they are worn again, some irritant in the pair of shoes may be suspected. Shoes are made of dozens of different materials, and scores of different chemicals are used in processing these materials. Identification of a specific irritant depends upon a PATCH TEST done with samples taken from the patient's shoes. The only remedy is to stop wearing a pair of shoes that gives trouble.

Show

A small amount or red or pink discharge from the vagina indicating the onset of labour.

Sickle cell anaemia

A hereditary abnormality of haemoglobin. Crises marked by

fever and attacks of pain occur.

A form of *pneumoconiosis*; chronic lung inflammation due to prolonged inhalation of dusts containing minute particles of iron.	**Siderosis**
S-shaped; especially, the *sigmoid flexure*, in the part of the colon above the rectum.	**Sigmoid**
Lung inflammation caused by inhalation of high concentrations of very fine particles of silicon over a period of time.	**Silicosis**
See PANHYPOPITUITARISM.	**Simmond's disease**
Nodules like calluses on the vocal cords of singers, orators, and others who use the voice to excess.	**Singer's nodes**
HICCUPS.	**Singultus**
A hollow space, cavity, recess, pocket, dilated channel, suppurating tract. Of the scores of medically designated sinuses, the *paranasal sinuses* – membrane-lined cavities in bones around the nose – are most familiar to laymen. *Sinusitis* (inflammation of the sinuses) is experienced to some degree by everyone who has a head cold, and more severly if drainage channels become blocked and congested and infection sets in.	**Sinus**
Transposition of all the organs of the chest and abdomen from the normal side of the body to the opposite side. For example, the liver is on the left side instead of the right. Total transposition does not necessarily impair general health.	**Situs inversus**
Application of wet heat to relieve pain, congestion, or spasm in the pelvic area, by sitting in a tub of warm water, 48°C(110°F) or more, which covers only the hips and buttocks.	**Sitz bath**
See DERMOGRAPHIA.	**Skin writing**

Sleep

New insight into sleep has come from studies with the ELECTROENCEPHALOGRAPH, but no one can yet say precisely what sleep is. Brain waves of experimental subjects show that we fall asleep in four stages, from Stage 1 (light sleep) to Stage 4 (deepest sleep), and awaken in reverse order. It takes about an hour and a half to go from light sleep to deep sleep and back again. There are about five such cycles in an average uninterrupted night's sleep of approximately eight hours. At the top, or light sleep phase of each cycle, we are close to waking, and may even wake and go back to sleep without remembering it. Perhaps this is the most critical time for insomniacs who fall asleep easily enough but wake in a little while and cannot get to sleep again. The discovery that dreaming is accompanied by a peculiar but characteristic kind of rapid eye movement has given some new information about dreams. Studies confirm that we generally have the first dream of the night after we ascend to light sleep from deep sleep. The average sleeper spends about two hours a night in dreams which occur in four or five cycles corresponding to light sleep. Experimenters believe that everybody dreams repeatedly every night but that dreams are almost immediately forgotten, remembered only if we awaken while a dream is in progress, and then not usually remembered for long.

Sleeping sickness
(*African trypanosomiasis*)

A disease with high fatality caused by organisms that get into the blood through the bites of tsetse flies indigenous to parts of Africa. It is not the same as sleepiness associated with some forms of encephalitis, which used to be called sleepy sickness.

Sleepwalking
(*somnambulism*)

Parents are often concerned about sleepwalking in children; the condition is less common in adults. Sleepwalkers may perform dangerous feats, but they also injure themselves by falling out of windows or crashing against objects. Anxiety and tension are often strong components of sleepwalking, and investigation of such factors is desirable if sleepwalking persists. The belief that it is dangerous to wake a sleepwalker has no basis in fact. It is better to wake him, to prevent injury to himself or others.

See RUPTURED DISC.	**Slipped disc**
A mass of dead tissue cast off from or contained in living tissue.	**Slough**
See VACCINIA.	**Smallpox vaccination**
Secretions or blood spread on a glass slide for examination under a microscope. Smears are often stained with various dyes to bring out the details of structure.	**Smears**
Thick whitish material that sometimes accumulates under the PREPUCE in men and around the CLITORIS in women.	**Smegma**

Snoring

The sounds of snoring are produced by vibrations of air passing in and out over the soft palate and other soft structures. Variations of sound are modified by the force of air flow, frequency of vibration, and the size, density, and elasticity of affected tissues. Sleeping on the back is conducive to snoring, but some people can snore while sleeping on their sides. A few causes of snoring may be correctable; it is worth consulting a doctor to find out. Most cases of snoring in children are associated with enlarged tonsils and adenoids. Snoring is often associated with mouth breathing, and if blocked nasal passages or predisposing conditions are treatable, the condition can be relieved. Nasal polyps are readily removed, a deviated septum can be corrected, blockages associated with infections and allergies are treatable. However, many snorers cannot be cured and often the best that can be done is to keep them from sleeping on their backs by sewing a rubber ball or something else uncomfortable, into the back of their pyjamas. The most practical remedy, useless to the snorer but of great value to his auditors, is ear plugs.

Soft contact lenses

Conventional contact lenses are made of optical glass or hard plastic. Soft lenses are made of water-absorbing plastic which stays soft and supple by absorbing moisture from the eye. Advantages claimed for soft lenses are: easier to fit (the lens moulds to the shape of the cornea); greater comfort; less chance of falling out (soft lenses cover about twice as much eye surface as hard ones). Disadvantages are: greater routine care (daily sterilization); inadequate correction of astigmatism; greater susceptibility to wear and damage; sometimes, alternate clearing and blurring of vision; higher cost. Progress in this field is rapid; improvement of materials and resolution of problems of sterilization are to be expected, as well as probable use of soft contacts as bandages for the eyes in certain conditions, and as carriers of medicines in conditions requiring frequent applications.

Solar urticaria	Nettle rash produced by exposure to sunlight.
Solitary kidney	A rare congenital condition; only one kidney is present.
Somatic	Of or relating to the body.
Somatotype	Body build, constitutional type. Somatotyping procedures most widely used today were developed by Dr. William H. Sheldon whose terms, *endomorph, mesomorph,* and *ectomorph* have entered the common medical language. Constitution-classifying is based on the three primitive cell layers of the embryo from which particular organs and systems develop. Skin and nervous system derive from the outside layer, the *ectoderm*. Bones, muscles and vascular system derive from the middle layer, the *mesoderm*. The lining of the gut derives from the inner layer, the *endoderm*. Everyone has all three components, but in varying proportions. The circus weight lifter, fat man, and living skeleton are extreme constitutional types. An extreme mesomorph has a predominance of muscle and bone and a hard, square build. An extreme endomorph has a good digestive tract, soft roundness of body, and great facility for getting fat. An extreme ectomorph with a preponderance of skin and nervous tissue has a slender build and great alertness to what is going on around him. Accurate somatotyping requires accurate measurements and photographing of the nude body.
Somniferous	Producing sleep.
Somniloquy (talking in sleep)	It is quite common for children to talk in their sleep. Even some adults worry that they may babble secrets when sleeping.

Words spoken in sleep are usually fragmentary, mumbled, even ludicrous, and probably indicate participation in dreams or remembered events of the previous day. Talking during sleep probably reflects decreased depth of sleep and is nothing to be alarmed about. See SLEEP.

Sudden, severe, involuntary contraction of muscles, interfering with function and often causing pain. If tightening of muscle is steady and persistent, as in leg cramps, it is called *tonic* spasm. If contractions alternate with relaxations, causing jerky movements, the spasms are called *clonic*. Both voluntary and involuntary muscles can be affected, causing a variety of *spastic* conditions. Spasms of involuntary muscle may involve the bronchial tubes (ASTHMA), intestines, blood vessels (RAYNAUD'S DISEASE), and sphincters of the gallbladder and urethra. Antispasmodic drugs such as belladonna may be prescribed to ease spastic conditions of involuntary muscle.	**Spasm**
A tubular instrument for viewing the interior of a passage or body cavity; for instance, the vagina, rectum, nose, ear.	**Speculum**
A swelling of the SCROTUM caused by cystic dilation (fluid-filled sac) of the sperm-conducting tubules of the testicle. Surgical removal of the painless cyst is usually desirable if it is persistent.	**Spermatocele**
An agent that kills SPERMATOZOA.	**Spermatocide**
Male germ cells; sperm. The sperm is the smallest human cell, and the only one capable of independent locomotion, by virtue of its tail. Sperms are produced in enormous numbers in the seminiferous tubules of the testicle. Primitive cells in the lining of the tubules develop into maturing sperms which fall off and are carried into a coiled tube, the *epididymis*, and thence into a straighter tube, the *vas deferens*. The journey takes about two weeks, during which the sperms continue to mature. The do not move under their own power until they are suspended in SEMEN at the time of ejaculation. Sperm production is a continuous process from puberty to old age. The average man	**Spermatozoa**

produces a vast number of sperms in his lifetime. The average ejaculate contains from 200 to 250 million sperms. An individual sperm has a head, neck, midpiece, and tail. The head carries the nucleus which contains 23 CHROMOSOMES, one of which is a sex chromosome – either an X (female-determining) of a Y (male-determining) chromosome. The sex chromosome of the human egg is always an X. Hence, it is the sperm that determines the sex of offspring. If the sperm contains a Y chromosome to pair with the X chromosome of the egg, the XY combination produces a boy. If the sperm contains an X chromosome to pair with the X of the egg, the combination produces a girl.

Sperm count	A laboratory procedure for estimating the number of SPERMATOZOA in a specimen of semen, useful in assessing male fertility. Although a count of 40,000,000 sperms per cubic centimetre of ejaculate is generally considered normal (counts two to three times greater are not unusual), conception can occur with a relatively low sperm population. Vigorous activity of sperms, and relative lack of abnormal forms, may be more significant to fertility than a relatively low sperm count. If sperms are vigorous and well-shaped, a sperm count of 20,000,000 per cubic centimetre is generally considered adequate for fertility. The volume of ejaculated semen ranges from two to six cubic centimetres.
Sphenoid	Wedge-shaped; especially, the bone which lies behind the upper part of the nasal cavity.
Sphincter	A muscle which surrounds and controls opening and closing of a natural orifice; for example, the anal sphincter.
Sphygmomanometer	The instrument used for measuring arterial blood pressure.
Spider (arterial)	Dilatation of small blood vessels in the skin, branching somewhat like the legs of a spider. Spider naevi may be associated with liver disease, pregnancy, varicose veins, and other conditions but may also occur in normal persons.
Spider bite	The BLACK WIDOW SPIDER, a common American spider, some-

times reaches the United Kingdom in fruit. Its bite is dangerous.

A congenital malformation of the spine in which some of the vertebrae fail to fuse, so that a sac containing the covers of the spinal cord and even the spinal cord itself may protrude under the skin.	**Spina bifida**
The soft column of nerve tissue enclosed in the vertebral column. *Spinal nerves* (all the nerves of the body except the twelve pairs of cranial nerves) enter or leave the spinal cord through openings in the vertebrae.	**Spinal cord**
A microbe shaped like a corkscrew. Many kinds of spirochaetes are harmless, but some cause syphilis, yaws, relapsing fever, tropical ulcer, ratbite fever, and other infections.	**Spirochaete**
Enlargement of the spleen.	**Splenomegaly**
A flap of skin from which the deeper layers have been cut away, leaving the outer layers for grafting.	**Split graft**
Inflammation of vertebrae.	**Spondylitis**
Deformation of the lower spine, due to the slipping forward of a lumber vertebra, usually on the sacrum.	**Spondylolisthesis**
A nail with a concave outer surface instead of the normal convexity, slightly resembling a spoon; often found in iron-deficiency anaemia.	**Spoon nail**
An inactive form of a microorganism that is resistant to destruction and capable of becoming active again. For example, TETANUS spores.	**Spore**
Infection by a kind of fungus that is parasitic on plants. The disease produces nodules along the course of lymphatic vessels which enlarge, ulcerate, and discharge pus. Nurserymen, farmers, and persons in contact with plants and woods are most susceptible. The infection is stubborn and may persist for months but usually responds to treatment.	**Sporotrichosis**

Spotting	A slight show of blood in the vaginal discharge at times other than menstruation. Slight spotting is not uncommon at the approximate time of OVULATION between menstrual periods. Spotting in pregnancy or after the menopause should be reported promptly to a doctor
Sprain	Tearing or laceration of ligaments that hold bones together at a joint, a result of severe wrenching. Sprains are sometimes difficult to distinguish from fractures; both may result from the same injury. Diagnosis should be left to the doctor.
Sprue	See MALABSORPTION SYNDROME.
Sputum	Matter which is coughed up from the lungs – that is, mucus and the substances entrapped in it.
Squint (*strabismus*)	Failure of the two eyes to direct their gaze simultaneously at the same object because of muscle imbalance.
S.R.N.	State-registered nurse.
Staghorn calculus	A large stone which more or less fills the pelvis of the kidney and has irregular projecting surfaces resembling antlers.
Stamp grafts	Small pieces of skin about the size of a postage stamp, used for grafting.
Stapes	A tiny stirrup-shaped bone of the middle ear. Fixation of the footplate of the stapes by bone growing around it (*otosclerosis*) prevents free conduction of sound to the inner ear. Several types of operations aim to correct this form of hearing loss. *Stapes mobilization* is a procedure to unfreeze the stirrup bone from its surroundings and restore free vibratory movements. In *stapedectomy*, the stirrup bone is replaced by a plastic substitute.
Staphylococci	Spherical bacteria which tend to grow in clumps like a bunch of grapes. They are common inhabitants of the skin and nasal passages.

S

Stagnation; slowing of normal flow of body fluids, blood, intestinal contents. **Stasis**

A severe, refractory condition. *Status asthmaticus*: intractable asthma, extreme dificulty in breathing, cyanosis, exhaustion, lasting a few days to a week or longer; *Status epilepticus*: epileptic attacks coming in rapid succession, during which the patient does not regain consciousness. **Status**

Stools containing large amounts of undigested fats. **Steatorrhoea**

A rare condition of sterility, absence of menstruation, and hairness, in women having enlarged ovaries with many cysts. Treatment is surgical removal of a wedge-shaped section of tissue from each ovary. **Stein-Leventhal syndrome**

Narrowing or constriction of a duct or aperture of the body. **Stenosis**

Any procedure which leaves a man or woman incapable of having children; usually, a surgical procedure. See TUBAL LIGATION and VASECTOMY. **Sterilization**

The breastbone. **Sternum**

Natural hormones or synthetic drugs whose molecules share a common basis of four rings of carbon atoms (the steroid nucleus) but which have different actions according to the attachment of other atoms. Natural steroids include the male and female sex hormones and cortisone-like hormones of the adrenal glands. Oral contraceptives (the pill) are steroids. Many synthetic steroids increase activity, enhance desired effects, minimize size effects, or otherwise improve the actions of a molecule by shifting, attaching, or detaching a few atoms. **Steroids**

An instrument which conducts bodily sounds, especially those of the heart, but of other organs as well, to the ears of the examiner. A piece of paper rolled into a cylinder, one end of which is placed on the chest of the patient and the other at the **Stethoscope** ear of the listener, demonstrates the principle. The stethoscope was invented by René Laennec, a French physician, in 1819.

Still's disease	A disease of children, like rheumatoid arthritis, affecting many different joints.
Stokes-Adams syndrome	Loss of consciousness, and sometimes convulsions, resulting from temporary cessation of the heartbeat in heart block. Nowadays the condition is often alleviated by the use of an electrical pacemaker.
Stomatitis	Inflammation of the mouth. The inflammation may be limited to the mouth or it may be a symptom of some systemic disease. Viruses, bacteria, or fungi may infect the mouth tissues, membranes may be sensitized to certain materials, some drugs may produce oral inflammation. Stomatitis may be an aspect of blood disorders, vitamin deficiencies, mechanical injuries from jagged teeth or ill-fitting dentures, and skin diseases. Treatment is as varied as the causes.
Stool	The bowel evacuation; faeces.
Strabismus	Squint.
Stratum corneum	The topmost horny layer of the outer skin or epidermis, composed of dead cells that are shed and replaced from below.
Strawberry mark	A birthmark comprised of superficial blood vessels, present at birth or developing shortly after, which has a tendency to disappear spontaneously.
Strawberry tongue	A bright red tongue seen especially in scarlet fever; the blood-engorged papillae are enlarged and prominent.
Streptococci	Bacteria which tend to grow like chains of little balls. They are responsible for scarlet fever, sore throat, and many other infections.

A streak, line, stripe, narrow band. Whitish striations of the abdomen may appear as the skin is stretched during pregnancy and in the breast after milk production ceases. Obesity or an excess of cortisone-like hormones may produce such marks on the abdomen. Striations may appear temporarily in adolescent girls as the sexual hormone balance is established.	**Stria** (pl. *striae*)
Narrowing or tightening of the passageway of a duct or hollow organ; may result from inflammation, contraction, injury, or scarring.	**Stricture**
Apoplexy, cerebrovascular accident.	**Stroke**
The supporting tissue of an organ, as opposed to its active, specific tissue.	**Stroma**
A cloth wrung out of hot water and applied to the skin; turpentine is sometimes sprinkled in the water as a counterirritant.	**Stupe**
An almost acute condition; intermediate between chronic and acute illness.	**Subacute**
A disease, usually mild, that has no definite symptoms or signs which can be recognized by the usual visual or clinical means.	**Subclinical disease**
Beneath the skin, as a hypodermic injection.	**Subcutaneous**
Partial or incomplete dislocation, sprain.	**Subluxation**
Underneath the breastbone.	**Substernal**
Sweat-inducing.	**Sudorific**
Prolonged unaccustomed exposure to intense sunlight will, as practically everyone has learned, cause sunburn, which is in every sense a burn. What most people want to acquire is a suntan, not a burn. The amount of sun that individuals can stand varies with thickness, pigmentation, and personal struc-	**Sunburn, suntan**

ture of the skin. The sun usually is intense enough to affect the skin between 9.30 a.m. and 4.30 p.m. from April to August. Of the ultraviolet rays: 5% are reflected off the skin surface, 65% absorbed by the horny layers of skin, 27% absorbed by the rest of the epidermis, 3% reach the dermis ('true skin"). To develop a tan without a burn, the skin should be exposed gradually, starting with an exposure of no more than twenty minutes on the first day, increasing exposure by about one third each successive day. After a week the skin should have been conditioned sufficiently to permit a moderate amount of sunbathing through the summer. Suntan is produced by the darkening and moving towards the surface of melanin granules made by cells in deeper skin layers. Exposure to sun not only darkens the skin, but thickens it. The extra thickness gives much of the protection against sunlight, but this thickness lasts only six weeks or so after exposure has ceased. Unlimited exposure to burning rays of the sun has undesirable long-term affects. Continued exposure ages the skin prematurely, thickening and wrinkling it.

Superfluous hair

Hirsutism; especially, excessive hairiness of the lips, cheek, chin, or legs of women, more obvious in brunettes. There may be an underlying endocrine disorder, a family tendency to hairiness, or hair may be unduly conspicuous in an area where it is not normally present. Electrolysis performed by a skilled operator employs electric current to destroy the hair root permanently, but its application is tedious. Chemical depilatories remove hair satisfactorily but directions must be followed carefully to avoid skin irritation. A bleach may mask the condition if hair growth is fine.

Supernumerary

More than the normal number, as a sixth finger or toe.

Suppuration

Formation of pus.

Suprarenal glands

Adrenal glands.

Supraspinatus syndrome

A term for disorders of the shoulder region which make it painful or impossible to lift the arm completely.

S

To sew up a wound, or the threadlike materials used for this purpose; catgut, linen, silk, wire, cotton, and so on. *Absorbable* sutures such as catgut are often used to close wounds in deep tissues. Sutures used to sew surface tissues are usually nonabsorbable and removable.	**Suture**
Athlete's foot of the ear canal; water incompletely drained from the ear sets up moist conditions favourable to fungus infection.	**Swimmer's ear**
Inflammatory disease of the hair follicles, especially of the beard. Usually a STAPHYLOCOCCAL infection, characterized by pus-filled pimples around hairs.	**Sycosis**
See CHOREA.	**Sydenham's chorea**
Surgical removal of fibres of the sympathetic nervous system.	**Sympathectomy**
Inflammation of one eye due to injury of the other eye. Prompt treatment of an injured eye is important to prevent involvement of the other eye and possible blindness.	**Sympathetic ophthalmia**
The junction of originally dictinct bones which have grown together; for example, the lines of fusion of the sacrum and the coccyx, and of the pubic bones.	**Symphysis**
Symptoms are subjective, that is, things of which the patient is aware, such as pain, stiffness, giddiness. Signs are objective, that is, things of which the patient is not aware, but the doctor finds, such as a heart murmur, a lump in the abdomen, or an absent reflex.	**Symptoms and signs**
A point of communication between the processes of nerve cells which come close together but do not actually touch.	**Synapse**
Fainting.	**Syncope**
Webbed or fused fingers or toes.	**Syndactyly**

Syndrome	A set of symptoms which occur together and collectively characterize a disease.
Synovial fluid	The clear fluid which lubricates the movements of tendons and joints.
Systemic disease	One which affects the body as a whole, not limited to a particular part; for example, an infection spread through the bloodstream.
Systole	The period of contraction of the heart. Systolic pressure is the higher of the two figures (such as 120/80) by which doctors express blood pressure readings. See DIASTOLE.

T

See ATAXIA.	**Tabes dorsalis**
Rapid heartbeat.	**Tachycardia**
TAPEWORM.	**Taenia**
Foot deformity; clubfoot.	**Talipes**
A plug of absorbent material inserted into a body cavity, such as a pack for nosebleed or a vaginal tampon to absorb menstrual flow.	**Tampon**
A ribbonlike flatworm which may invade the intestines of consumers of undercooked beef, fish, or pork.	**Tapeworm**
Emptying fluids from a body cavity by surgical puncture; resorted to when accumulated fluids affect the functioning of the heart, lungs, abdomen, or other organs.	**Tapping**
The instep of the foot.	**Tarsus**
Hard, mineralized deposits on the surface of teeth, irritating to the gums and underlying bone. Toothbrushing helps to prevent the deposits when they are in the soft state, but they solidify quickly. Periodic removal by a dentist is good insurance against disease of supporting tissues of the teeth, popularly called pyorrhoea.	**Tartar** (*dental calculus*)
Insertion of permanent colours into the skin through punctures, as by a needle. Unsterilized tattoo needles can transmit viral HEPATITIS and other diseases. In competent medical hands, tattooing has recognized but limited value, primarily for minimizing skin discolorations. *Portwine stain*, a bluish-red birthmark, may be made less conspicuous by tattooing opaque skin-coloured pigments into the affected area.	**Tattooing**
A hereditary disease occurring mostly in Jewish children, manifested early in infancy, characterized by muscle weakness and blindness. With an ophthalmoscope a characteristic bright cherry spot can be seen at the back of the infant's eye. No	**Tay-Sachs disease**

known treatment can reverse the condition and life expectancy is short. Certain related diseases which occur later in life do not have a racial incidence.

Telangiectasis

Dilatation of groups of small blood vessels, appearing as fine red or blue lines on the skin, sometimes associated with diseases of the skin, cirrhosis of the liver, and other disorders. The dilatations may form hard, red, wartlike spots te size of a pinhead or pea. In *hereditary haemorrhagic telangiectasis*, a rare form, the dilated vessels become thin and fragile, rupture spontaneously, and bleed into the skin, intestines, or other parts of the body. It is inherited as a dominant trait.

Temporomandibular joint

The joint in front of the ear in which the hinge of the lower jaw fits into a socket in the base of the skull. Its close relationship to the teeth may bring about changes not common in other joints. Uneven bite, tooth-clenching habits, poorly fitting dentures, or tooth restorations may limit sideways motion, limit the opening of the mouth, cause pain, soreness, clicking noises, and even headaches.

Tendinitis

Inflammation of tendons and their attachments.

Tendon

A band or cord of tough white fibrous tissue that connects a muscle to a bone. Muscle fibres merge into one end of a tendon, the other end of which is attached to a bone. Sometimes a tendon conveys muscle action over a considerable distance, as in the back of the leg, where a long tendon inserted into the rear of the ankle transmits the pull of calf muscles above it. This makes it unnecessary to have a huge mass of muscle around the ankle itself. Most tendons are covered by sheaths which secrete lubricating fluid for easy sliding. Tendons and their sheaths are subject to injury by tearing, stretching, twisting stresses (pulled tendon is a common athletic injury) and to inflammations, for which there are technical names such as *tenosynovitis* and *tenovaginitis*.

Tenesmus

Painful straining to empty the bowel, without success.

Tennis elbow

This painful condition of the outer side of the elbow joint can affect anyone who overvigorously uses a screwdriver as well as a tennis racket. It is a form of BURSITIS produced by violent extension of the wrist with the palm downward or vigorous rotary movement of the forearm against resistance, putting severe stress on the elbow joint.

The branch of science concerned with the study of malformations. A *teratoma* is a tumour containing hair, teeth, bones, or other material not normal to the part in which it grows.	**Teratology**
The end of the normal period of gestation or pregnancy when birth occurs.	**Term (at term)**
The primary male sex glands or gonads; paired organs, enclosed in the SCROTUM, together with accessory structures.	**Testicles, testes**
The male sex hormone, a STEROID hormone produced by cells of the testicle independent from cells which produce SPERMATOZOA.	**Testosterone**
A serious infection caused by toxins of tetanus organisms which get into the body through perforating, penetrating, or deep wounds and thrive in the absence of oxygen. The main features are violent spasms of muscles. The disease is easily prevented by *tetanus toxoid* injections. These are routinely given to infants and should be just as routine for adults.	**Tetanus (lockjaw)**
Painful muscle spasms, especially of wrists and feet; sometimes convulsions. Insufficient calcium in the blood causes the muscular irritability and consequent symptoms. Insufficiency of circulating calcium may result from vitamin D deficiency or underactivity of the parathyroid glands. Treatment is with calcium salts, orally or by infusion if the condition is severe. Not to be confused with TETANUS.	**Tetany**
Congenital malformation of the heart, exhibiting four defects: aorta turned to the right, ventricular septal defect, constriction of the pulmonary artery or valve, hypertrophy of the right ventricle.	**Tetralogy of Fallot**

Thalassaemia	A congenital form of anaemia which occurs primarily in people native to Mediterranean countries or their descendants.
Therapy	Treatment of disease. Anything that is therapeutic is designed to help or heal.
Thermography	Body surfaces emit slightly different amounts of heat because of local differences in underlying blood supply. This is the principle of thermography, which employs sensitive instruments to scan body areas and record slight heat differentials. Thermography has been used to detect and localize very small breast tumours, to investigate blood vessel obstructions, and to localize the site of the placenta.
Thoracentesis	Puncture of the chest wall with a hollow needle for withdrawal of fluid.
Thorax	The chest.
Threadworms	Small roundworms which may infest the intestines, usually in children.
Thrombin	An enzyme present in blood oozing from a wound, but not in circulating blood. It acts upon a blood protein to produce *fibrin*, which is the essential portion of a blood clot.
Thromboangiitis obliterans	See BUERGER'S DISEASE
Thrombocytes	Blood PLATELETS, which help to initiate blood clotting.
Thrombocytopenia	Deficiency of platelets necessary for blood coagulation, resulting in bleeding from tiny blood vessels into the skin and mucous membranes, known as PURPURA.
Thrombophlebitis	Presence of a blood clot (THROMBUS) in a vein, with inflammation; *venous thrombosis*. Veins of the leg are most commonly affected. If superficial, the affected vein may be felt as a tender cord. Thrombosis of deep veins is serious because blood clots may break off and be carried in the bloodstream until they plug

vital vessels. A large piece (EMBOLUS) may reach the lungs and cause death. The tendency of clots to form in slightly injured veins is greatly increased by physical inactivity such as prolonged bed rest. Getting the patient out of bed soon after surgery or childbirth, and encouraging bedridden patients to carry out frequent movements of the legs, are preventive measures. Treatment of active deep venous thrombosis includes such measures as elevation of the foot of the bed, warmth, and anticoagulant drugs which retard blood clotting.

Formation of a clot in a blood vessel, and the partial or complete plugging of the vessel that ensues. The most familiar example is *coronary thrombosis*, but the process can occur in many vessels besides those which supply the heart. **Thrombosis**

A clot which forms in a blood vessel and remains at the site of attachment. If a fragment or the entire clot breaks off and is carried through the bloodstream, it is called an EMBOLUS. **Thrombus**

See CANDIDIASIS. **Thrush**

An organ in the chest which for years puzzled anatomists who could find no function for it. Recent research has shown that immediately after birth, the thymus begins to activate the body's defences against infections. The thymus produces and sends out millions of *lymphocytes* to the spleen and lymph nodes, where they synthesize ANTIBODIES. Once these seedbeds are established with the aid of a hormone from the thymus, production of lymphocytes in lymphoid tissues continues throughout life. The thymus then shrinks. In infants the thymus is a large organ, relative to body size. It continues to grow for eight to ten years. By that time the body's immunity systems are running smoothly and the thymus is no longer necessary. The gland begins to shrink and in adults is very small. At one time it was thought that an enlarged thymus was a cause of sudden unexplained deaths of infants, because the thymus of infants dead from infections was much smaller than the thymus of infants who died suddenly from unknown causes. It is now realized that the thymus of infants who die **Thymus gland** from infections is abnormally small because the gland shrinks rapidly in the presence of infections and stresses, and that a relatively large thymus is normal in infancy.

Thyroglobulin

An iodine-protein substance, the form in which thyroid hormone is stored in the gland.

Thyroid

The shield-shaped gland in the neck, covering the front and sides of the windpipe. It is a regulator of metabolism, the rate at which the body burns its fuel.

Thyroidectomy

Surgical removal of part of the thyroid gland.

Thyroiditis

Acute or chronic inflammation of the thyroid gland.

Thyrotoxicosis

Hyperthyroidism; a toxic condition due to excessive activity of the thyroid gland, or to a tumour of the gland.

Thyroxine

The hormone released from the thyroid gland.

Tibia

The larger and more prominent of the two bones in the lower leg.

Tic douloureux
(*trigeminal neuralgia*)

Stabbing, excruciating pain in one side of the face along the course of the fifth cranial nerve, set off by touching a trigger area.

Tics

Habit spasms; quick, repetitive movements of certain muscle groups, always in the same manner: pouting the lips, blinking the eyelids, wrinkling the nose, making faces, shaking the head, shrugging a shoulder, tilting the neck, and so on. These nervous habits develop most commonly in children and often disappear in the course of time if the child is not nagged about them. Usually the child is tense to begin with; he may be a target of excessive demands, expectations, and pressures. A little loosening of the reins by those who hold them may help to relax a child who, after all, does not consciously decide to indulge in tics. Nervous habits should be distinguished from purposeless movements associated with some physical disorder. Genuine tics never appear during sleep.

Three times a day.	**T.i.d.**
Ringworm; fungus infection of the skin.	**Tinea**
Ringworm of the groin; a fungus infection of the skin of the upper thighs near the genital organs. It is caused by the same group of organisms responsible for athlete's foot. Because the symptoms are similar to those of psoriasis and other skin diseases, a doctor should be consulted. It is easily cured.	**Tinea cruris** (*Dhobi itch*)
A form of TUBERCULIN TEST. A small disposable stainless steel disc with four prongs covered with dried *tuberculin* is pressed into the skin. The unit is used on only one patient, never reused. The technique is advantageous in screening large population groups of school children and susceptible young adults for tuberculosis.	**Tine test**
Head noises; ringing, roaring, clicking, or hissing sounds in the ears.	**Tinnitus**
Forward, backward, or other displacement of the uterus from its normal position.	**Tipped uterus**
A method of growing cells in a suitable nutrient in flasks or test tubes outside the body, and of propagating viruses in the cells. Polio viruses and some others are grown in tissue culture for manufacture of vaccines. Viruses can be identified by tissue-culture reactions under laboratory conditions. More than 100 new viruses have been isolated and identified by tissue culture techniques in the past decade and some have been associated with diseases.	**Tissue culture**
Ability to withstand abnormally large doses of a drug, induced by its continual use.	**Tolerance**
X-ray films of layers or planes of the body. A tomogram shows a plane of the body about a half inch thick. The layer shows fine detail but structures above and below it are blurred.	**Tomograms**
An instrument for measuring the pressure in the eyeball, used	**Tonometer**

in screening for *glaucoma*.

Tophi

Urate deposits in the external ear, joints, and other structures composed largely of CARTILAGE; characteristic of *gout*.

Torticollis (*wryneck*)

A condition in which the muscles of one side of the neck are in a state of more or less continuous spasm, pulling the head into an unnatural position.

Toxaemia

A poisoned condition due to absorption into the blood of toxic substances produced by bacteria or body cells, but without the presence of bacteria in the blood. *Toxaemia of pregnancy* is a disturbance of metabolism which in severe form (rare if the patient has good prenatal care) is attended by fever, headache, convulsions, and a rapid rise in blood pressure.

Toxic goitre

THYROTOXICOSIS, hyperthyroidism.

Toxin

A poisonous substance originating in microbes, animals, or plants. Injection of a specific toxin into an animal stimulates the production of specific ANTIBODIES. This is the basis for pharmaceutical preparation of an antitoxin that neutralizes a particular toxin, for example: *botulinus, tetanus, diphtheria, snake venom*.

Toxoid

Resembling a toxin; a substance prepared by treating a toxin with agents which produce a *toxoid* that has the same immunity-stimulating ability as the toxin but is itself harmless and nontoxic. Tetanus and diphtheria toxoids are widely used in routine immunization.

Toxoplasmosis

A disease caused by infection with protozoan organisms. Inapparent infection of a pregnant woman may cause severe abnormalities in her baby.

Tracer elements

See RADIOISOTOPES.

Trachea

The windpipe.

Tracheobronchitis

Inflammation of the windpipe and bronchial tubes.

T

Cutting a hole in the windpipe to bypass an obstruction and permit air to flow into the lungs.

Tracheotomy

A contagious disease of the eyes, caused by viruses which attack the lining membranes of the lids and eyes, leading to ulcers and blindness.

Trachoma

A popular, nonmedical term for a variety of drugs which more or less selectively depress the central nervous system to produce calming, sedative effects but which, in proper doses, do not dull consciousness or induce sleep. Tranquillizer is a broad term that includes many drugs of somewhat different individual actions. The drugs are often categorized as *major* and *minor* tranquillizers. The major tranquillizers, most of which belong to chemical families known as *phenothiazines* and *piperazines*, have their greatest use in treating severely disturbed psychotic patients. They tend to reduce agitation, excitement, panic, and hostility, and to quiet the wild destructive behaviour associated with those emotional states, and there may be a reduction of psychotic symptoms such as hallucinations and delusions. This often makes the calmed patient more receptive of and amenable to other forms of therapy. Many patients must continue on the drugs for varying lengths of time, but this often can be supervised by the doctor, and recovery tends to be assisted by a comfortable home and family environment. The major tranquillizers are sometimes used in nonpsychiatric patients for their secondary actions in preventing or arresting nausea and vomiting, and for intensifying the actions of anaesthetics and pain-relievers so that smaller doses of the latter can be given. The minor tranquillizers (sometimes called *ataractics*) are mainly used to suppress mild to moderate manifestations of anxiety and tension in psychoneurotic patients as well as in normal persons who react tensely to stress of their environment. Their action is similar to, and probably not superior to, that of the hypnotics in easing anxiety-tension states. However, the classic sedatives cause some drowsiness and loss of alertness; in correct doses, the minor tranquillizers produce mild sedation without dulling consciousness or impairing performance. Some of them have moderate muscle-relaxing action. The minor tranquillizers

Tranquillizers

have a considerably greater margin of safety than potent sedatives, and massive overdosage is less likely to be serious or fatal, although huge overdoses, taken with suicidal intent, can lead to coma, collapse, and even death. Patients who take excessive amounts of the drugs for long periods may become dependent upon them and suffer withdrawal reactions when they are discontinued.

Transillumination

Examination of a cavity or structure by means of light passing through it; for example, examination of nasal sinuses with a light in the patient's mouth.

Transplantation

Surgical techniques for transplanting an organ from one person to another are well advanced. The best known procedure is kidney transplantation, but the heart, lung, liver, and spleen have occasionally been transplanted, demonstrating that surgical techniques of transplantation have been mastered. The major obstacle to permanent transplantation is the body's ultimate rejection of a donated organ as foreign tissue by the patient's immune mechanisms.

Transvestism

Desire to wear the clothes of the opposite sex; a person who does so is a *transvestite*.

Trauma

Injury, wound.

Tremor

Involuntary quivering and trembling of muscle groups, other than from obvious causes such as shivering from cold. Tremor is a symptom which may give information about a constitutional disease. A doctor may ask a patient to hold out the arms at shoulder level with palms down and fingers stretched; fine, rapid tremor of the fingers may suggest hyperthyroidism. There are fine, coarse, slow, and rapid tremors; harmless hereditary tremors; tremors that appear when at rest; and intention tremor that appears when voluntary movement of a part is attempted. Tremors may or may not indicate a disorder of the nervous system; there are hysterical tremors that have no organic basis.

Trench fever

A louse-borne, typhus-like RICKETTSIAL INFECTION. Many

T

cases occurred in World Wars I and II but the disease has since disappeared.

Painful, swollen, malodorous inflammation of the mouth and gums. The disease is not considered to be contagious. Susceptibility is increased by malnutrition, poor mouth hygiene, and heavy smoking.	**Trench mouth** (*Vincent's infection*)
Cutting a circular section of bone out of the skull with a *trephine*, an instrument with sawlike edges.	**Trepanning**
A kind of corkscrew-shaped microbe responsible for a number of infectious diseases, including syphilis.	**Treponema**
The muscle that extends the forearm.	**Triceps**
A parasitic disease due to ingestion of encysted larvae of worms present in raw or undercooked pork.	**Trichinosis** (*trichiniasis*)
A ball of hair formed in the stomach.	**Trichobezoar**
A common infestation of the vagina with minute pearshaped protozoa. Their presence produces vaginal irritation and a thin, white, watery, offensive discharge. Men may also be infected but often have no symptoms. Local methods of treatment by insufflation of powders, medicated douches, and so on give relief but the organisms are hard to eradicate. Infection may be retransmitted by marital partners and for total eradication, both partners may be treated. A new oral drug, *metronidazole*, is highly effective in eradicating the infection.	**Trichomoniasis**
Ringworm of the scalp. The causative fungi fluoresce when exposed to ultraviolet light. The condition, which is contagious, occurs in children before puberty.	**Trichophytosis**
A valve with three triangular-shaped leaflets through which blood moves from atrium to ventricle in the right side of the heart.	**Tricuspid valve**

Trigeminal neuralgia	See TIC DOULOUREUX.
Trigger finger	A condition in which efforts to unbend a finger are at first unsuccessful, but it soon straightens with a snap or a jerk, like the release of a trigger. It is caused by a constriction which prevents free movement of a tendon in its sheath.
Trimester	Three months, or one third of the nine months of pregnancy. The nine months of pregnancy are traditionally divided into the first, second, and third trimesters.
Triple vaccine	Vaccine combining immunizing agents against *diphtheria*, *pertussis* (whooping cough), and *tetanus*, administered in a single injection instead of separate injections for each disease.
Trismus	Spasmodic tightening of muscles of the jaw, as in lockjaw (tetanus).
Trocar	A perforating instrument for puncturing a cavity to release fluid; it fits inside a *cannula*.
Tropical ulcer	Chronic, tissue-destroying ulceration of the lower leg or foot, caused by a spirochaete.
Truss	A device, usually a pad attached to a belt, designed to hold in place a HERNIA or internal organ which tends to protrude.
Trypanosomiasis	African sleeping sickness, produced by organisms transmitted to the blood by the bite of an infected insect.
Tryptophane	One of the essential AMINO ACIDS. It is frequently inadequate in food protein of plant origin.
TSH	Thyroid-stimulating hormone.
Tsutsugamushi disease	See SCRUB TYPHUS
Tubal ligation (*salpingectomy*)	An operation for sterilization of women. The surgeon makes a small incision in the abdomen and cuts and ties the FAL-

LOPIAN TUBES. This prevents the meeting of sperm and egg and makes conception impossible. The procedure is comparable in severity to an appendix operation and is always performed in hospital. It is frequently performed a few hours after delivery of a baby but can be done at any time for a nonpregnant woman. Tubal ligation does not interfere with menstruation or sexual capacity; the ovaries continue to produce hormones. It is important to regard the sterilization as permanent, but restoration of fertility can sometimes be achieved by a further operation. A recent development entails nipping the tubes with a plastic clip or ring, instead of severing them. This procedure damages the tube less, so that if fertility is desired there is a better chance of this being achieved. It must always be understood that no surgeon, however skilful, can guarantee to re-establish fertility. The operation is often done with a laparoscope – that is, a special telescope which is passed through the abdominal wall.

Implantation of a fertilized egg in the walls of the Fallopian tube instead of in the uterus; the most common form of ECTOPIC PREGNANCY.	**Tubal pregnancy**
A small nodule or prominence; especially, a mass of small spherical cells produced by tubercle bacilli that is characteristic of tuberculosis. The word also means a small rounded prominence on a bone.	**Tubercle**
A skin test for tuberculosis. Tuberculin in various forms is a sterile fluid containing substances extracted from dead tuberculosis germs. Tissues of a person with tuberculous infection are sensitive to products of tubercle bacilli. Injection of a small amount of tuberculin under the skin gives a positive or negative reaction. A positive reaction, indicated by redness and swelling of the injected area within a few hours, indicates the presence of tuberculous infection but does not tell whether the infection is old or new, active or inactive. It merely indicates that tuberculous infection was acquired at some time.	**Tuberculin test**
A little tube; any minute tubular structure, such as the kidney	**Tubule**

	tubules or the seminiferous tubules of the testes.
Tumefaction	Swelling.
Turbinates	Scroll-shaped bones of the outer walls of the nasal cavity, covered by spongy tissue which warms, moistens, and filters inhaled air.
Turner's syndrome	A congenital condition in which the ovaries neither mature nor produce egg cells. The affected girl develops along female lines but breast enlargement and menstruation do not occur at puberty, unless the condition is recognized early and treated with female hormones; however, the patient is permanently sterile. A woman with Turner's syndrome has only 45 instead of the normal 46 CHROMOSOMES. One sex chromosome is missing. A normal woman has two XX (female) chromosomes; in Turner's syndrome, one X chromosome is lack. Its absence results in ovaries lacking egg-producing follicles, and there is retardation of body growth; ultimate adult height is usually less than five feet.
Tussis	Cough.
Twins	See MULTIPLE BIRTHS.
Tympanoplasty	Plastic surgery of the middle ear to clean out and reconstruct the cavity.
Tympanum	The eardrum, the *tympanic membrane*.
Typhoid fever	Acute feverish illness caused by germs of the salmonella family, contained in the faeces of infected patients and unknowing carriers; usually transmitted by contaminated water or food or poor personal hygiene. Modern sanitation, alert health departments, and medical progress have made typhoid fever a rare disease where it was once common, feared, disabling, and often deadly. An antibiotic, chloramphenicol, is effective in treating typhoid fever. Vaccination against the disease (three inoculations a week or more apart, and an annual booster dose if one remains in an infected area) is recommended for travel-

lers to regions where typhoid fever is endemic.

A RICKETTSIAL DISEASE transmitted to man by infected lice and fleas, with rats and mice as intermediaries. There are several varieties of typhus. The disease is endemic in parts of Asia, the near East, India, and other areas. Vaccination is recommended for travellers to such areas.

Typhus

An open sore with an inflamed base; local disintegration of tissues of the skin or mucous membranes, leaving a raw, sometimes running surface. The cause may be infection, pressure (as in PRESSURE SORES), erosive irritation (PEPTIC ULCER), varicosities, systemic disease, impaired circulation.	**Ulcer**
Inflammation of the colon and rectum, characterized by ulcers inside the tube and blood-streaked diarrhoea. The disease may be mild and responsive to medical treatment or so severe as to require surgical removal of the affected part of the colon.	**Ulcerative colitis**
The bone on the side of the forearm opposite to the thumb; its companion bone is the radius.	**Ulna**
Sound waves of high frequencies above the range of human hearing. Ultrasonic devices have several medical uses. Instruments which register the echoes of ultrasound have been used to locate and define brain tumours, to locate the position of the placenta and fetus, and to identify the site and severity of arterial obstruction by registering the rate of blood flow in deep vessels. Therapeutically, ultrasonic equipment is used to clean tartar from teeth, to treat bursitis, and an ultrasound probe has had some success in destroying nerve endings in the inner ear, without damage to hearing and the sense of equilibrium, in patients with Ménière's disease who have not responded to medical treatment.	**Ultrasound**
Wavelengths of radiation too short to be seen as visible light. They lie between the wavelengths of visible light and X-rays. The spectrum of visible light runs from short violet rays to long red rays. The sequence of colours in a rainbow or sunlight scattered by a prism is violet, indigo, blue, green, yellow, orange, red. Beyond red lie the long invisible *infrared rays*, sometimes used to deliver dry heat to parts of the body. Ultraviolet rays contained in sunshine or produced by ultraviolet lamps (sunlamps) act upon substances in the skin to make vitamin D. They also produce a skin tan (see SUNBURN). These are the only known benefits of ultraviolet rays in moderation. Excessive exposure to natural or artificial ultraviolet radiation can produce burns, and age the skin prema-	**Ultraviolet rays**

turely. It is wise to ask for and follow a doctor's advice on the use of sunlamps.

Umbilical cord

The long flexible cord which is attached to the PLACENTA at one end and to the abdomen of the fetus at the other. It is the lifeline of the fetus. Through vessels of the cord the fetus receives nutrients and disposes of wastes. The cord allows considerable freedom of movement in the womb. The cord continues to function until it is tied and severed at birth.

Umbilical hernia

A protrusion of the intestines through a weakness in the abdominal wall in the region of the navel, not uncommon in infants.

Umbilicated

Depressed like a navel.

Umbilicus

The navel, belly-button; a depressed round scar in the middle of the abdomen, a reminder of the umbilical vessels that once nourished the fetus by the placenta.

Uncinaria

HOOKWORMS.

Underweight

Body weight ten per cent less than desirable weight is usually considered to be underweight. However, healthy people vary in bone and muscle proportions and rates of energy expenditure. Underweight may be a symptom of some disease process and should be evaluated by a doctor; sudden unexplained loss of weight requires medical investigation.

Undescended testicles

See CRYPTORCHIDISM.

Undulant fever

See BRUCELLOSIS.

Uniovular

Of or relating to or originating from a single egg, as identical twins.

Universal donor

A person with Type O blood does not have factors which would antagonize the blood of Types A, B, or AB, and hence is presumably compatible with all blood types. However, there are many blood factors besides the ABO group (Rh, M, N,

Lewis, Kell, Duffy, Lutheran, and others) which may make the blood of a Type O donor antagonistic to a recipient. A universal donor's blood may be given in an emergency, but cross-matching of blood is necessary for greatest safety in transfusions.

See POLYUNSATURATED FATS.   **Unsaturated fats**

Infection of nasal passages or throat above the lungs. An   **Upper respiratory**
infection may extend from the original site of symptoms.   **infection**

Presence in the blood of toxic substances due to incapacity of   **Uraemia**
the kidney to filter and excrete them in urine; *uraemic poisoning*. Symptoms may develop in a few hours or over a period
of weeks: headache, dimness of vision, drowsiness, restlessness;
later, diarrhoea and vomiting, difficult breathing during the
night, convulsions, coma, death. It is the way in which serious
kidney disease usually terminates.

A nitrogen-containing substance in blood and urine, formed   **Urea**
mainly from nitrogen groups removed in the liver from the
AMINO ACIDS of protein foods. Some is formed from nitrogen
released by the wear and tear of body tissues. Increasing the
protein portion of the diet increases the output of urea in the
urine. The *urea clearance test* of blood is a test of kidney
function.

The narrow tube through which urine from the kidneys passes   **Ureter**
into the bladder. Urine is not drawn down the tube by gravity,
nor does it descend in a steady flow. The ureter has walls of
smooth muscle which contract in waves (PERISTALSIS) to move
urine into the bladder in jets which occur a few times a
minute.

The canal from the neck of the bladder to the outside, through   **Urethra**
which urine is passed. The female urethra is about 4 cm
(1½ in) long; the male urethra, 20 to 23 cm (8 to 9 in).
Voiding of urine is regulated by circularly arranged sphincter
muscles which in the adult are largely under voluntary control.

Urethritis	Inflammation of the URETHRA.

Uric acid	A nitrogen-containing compound present in normal blood and urine. It is derived from substances in the nuclei of cells called *purines,* in which liver, sweetbreads, kidney, and other glandular meats are rich. An excess of uric acid-products is characteristic of GOUT, a disorder in which tiny urate crystals tend to be deposited in cartilage and cause pain.

Uricaemia	Excessive amounts of URIC ACID in the blood.

Urinalysis	Inspection and chemical analysis of urine. The extent of analysis depends on what the doctor wants to find out. At the minimum, observations of colour, clarity, specific gravity, acidity, sugar, and ALBUMIN content are usually made. More extensive microscopic or chemical analysis of possible constituents – pus, bile, blood cells, crystals, casts – may be neccessary to throw light on what is going on in the body.

Urine	The amber-coloured, slightly acid fluid secreted by the kidneys. It is mostly water but normally contains about four per cent of dissolved materials such as salt, ammonia, urea, uric acid, hormones or their breakdown products, and pigments. Excessive or deficient amounts of normal constituents may indicate disease, and abnormal constituents – fat, blood, pus, bacteria, spermatozoa, bile – almost always do. Acidity of the urine varies with the diet. Most fruits reduce the activity of the diet; starvation or a high protein diet increases it. Acidity of the urine indicates that the kidneys are doing their job of maintaining the slight alkalinity of the blood (see ACID-BASE BALANCE). The average adult forms about 1.5l ($2\frac{1}{7}$ pints) or urine a day. The volume of urine is reduced in hot weather, by strenuous muscular exercise or scanty fluid intake, and is greater on a high than a low protein diet. The most concentrated urine is passed after getting up in the morning. Doctors have good reason for specifying that a sample of urine should be taken at a certain time. Formation of urine is decreased during sleep; decided and persistent increase of volume of night urine may be a sign of chronic kidney or other disease. The yellow pigment that gives urine its colour is called *urochrome.*

See GENITOURINARY.	**Urogenital**

A medical specialist in diseases of the urinary tract in females and of the genitourinary tract in male patients. **Urologist**

FALLOPIAN TUBES. **Uterine tubes**

X-rays of the uterus and tubes, after injection of iodized oil to determine whether or not the tubes are open. **Uterosalpingography**

Uterus

The womb; the pear-shaped, muscular, hollow, distensible home of the fetus in pregnancy. In the adult nonpregnant woman the uterus is about 7.5 cm (3 in) long, 6 cm (2 $\frac{1}{}$ in) wide near the top, tapering to a neck (*cervix*) about 2.5 cm (1 in) wide, which occupies the upper part of the vagina. The uterus has walls of smooth muscle with a lining of mucous membrane (endometrium). Its triangular cavity is continuous with a narrow canal through its neck which affords an entrance for SPERMATOZOA and an exit for menstrual discharges. The uterus lies between the bladder and the rectum, tilted forward, its upper part resting on the bladder. It is loosely supported by eight LIGAMENTS which allow freedom of motion and position in adjusting to pressures of surrounding organs and enlargement in pregnancy. The organ enlarges slightly during menstruation, enormously during pregnancy, and after childbirth returns almost to its previous size, but its cavity is larger than before.

Uvea

Pigmentary layers of the eye: the IRIS, CILIARY BODY, and CHOROID coat, composed largely of interlaced blood vessels vital to the eye's nutrition.

Uveitis

Inflammation of the UVEA, and associated eye structures. It is a serious condition that can cause blindness. It may be associated with systemic diseases (TOXOPLASMOSIS, HISTOPLASMOSIS, LEPTOSPIROSIS), but there are many types of uveal inflammation for which no specific cause can be found. One form is thought to be an AUTO-IMMUNE DISEASE resulting from a patient's sensitization to tissues of the lens of his own eyes.

Uvula

The blob of tissue hanging from the soft palate at the back of the mouth. It can be seen with a mirror by opening the mouth wide and depressing the tongue. It rarely causes any trouble, except that it may be implicated in snoring.

Vaccine

The word derives from the Latin word for cow, the source of cowpox virus used to vaccinate against smallpox. It has come to mean any bacterial or viral material for inoculation against a specific disease. Virus vaccines are of two types, *live virus* or *killed virus* vaccines. Live virus vaccines contain living viruses, so weakened that they cannot cause significant disease, but can still stimulate the body powerfully to make protective ANTI-BODIES against a particular disease. Killed virus vaccines contain viruses treated by physical or chemical means to kill or inactivate them so that they cannot cause disease but nevertheless can stimulate immunity-producing mechanisms of the body. In general, live virus vaccines are more potent and create longer lasting immunity than killed virus vaccines.

Vaccinia

Cowpox; a disease of cattle caused by a virus which, inoculated into man, creates immunity to smallpox. Babies used to be vaccinated against smallpox before they were a year old but routine vaccination is no longer recommended (infants with eczema, impetigo, or skin rashes should not be vaccinated until the condition clears up, nor should they be in close contact with others who have just been vaccinated). About three days after smallpox vaccination a red pimple appears at the site of inoculation, enlarges, becomes a blister, and is surrounded by a reddened area. The lesion begins to dry in a week to ten days. It forms a scab which falls off by the end of the third week or sooner, leaving a flat whitish mark. Reaction to one's first smallpox vaccination is known as a primary take. Reactions in persons who have been vaccinated previously are milder, but if there is no reaction at all it does not necessarily mean that one is naturally immune, but that the vaccine was weak or did not get through the skin. Smallpox is now a very rare disease.

Vacuole

A clear space in tissue.

Vacuum extractor
(ventous)

A cuplike device within which a partial vacuum is created when it is placed over the presenting part of a baby's head during childbirth. The adherent cup with its handle facilitates extraction of the baby and the device is sometimes used in delivery as a substitute for obstetric forceps.

Vagina	A sheath; the female organ of copulation, a muscular canal lined with mucous membrane which opens at the surface of the body and extends inward to the cervix of the uterus.
Vaginal diaphragm	A contraceptive device consisting of a spring-rimmed rubber dome inserted into the vagina to cover the cervix.
Vaginal hysterectomy	Surgical removal of the uterus through the vagina.
Vaginismus	Painful spasm of the female pelvic muscles, making sexual intercourse difficult or impossible.
Vaginitis	Inflammation of the vagina, characterized by discharge and discomfort; see CANDIDIASIS and TRICHOMONIASIS. A form occurring after the menopause is called *atrophic* or *senile vaginitis.*
Vagotomy	Cutting of certain branches of the VAGUS nerve. The object is to diminish the flow of nerve impulses, such as those which stimulate the stomach to produce acid.
Vagus	The tenth cranial nerve which arises in the brain and extends its fibres to the pacemaker of the heart, to the bronchi, oesophagus, gallbladder, pancreas, small intestine, and secretory glands of the stomach.
Valsalva manoeuvre	Originally a technique devised by an Italian anatomist for pushing air into the middle ear by exhaling forcibly while keeping the glottis closed. A similar condition is produced by coughing or straining when passing a stool. The manoeuvre is used by cardiologists as a diagnostic test of congestive heart failure. Increase of pressure in the chest and abdomen prevents the return flow of blood from the head, hands, and feet. Heart output decreases and venous blood pressure increases. When the effort is ended, a surge of venous blood into the right side of the heart causes temporary overloading of the heart chambers. The mechanism explains why some persons feel light-headed or dizzy during bowel movements or while coughing.

V

A structure that prevents backflow of fluids. There are valves in the heart, in many veins, at the stomach outlet, and at junctions along many tubes, to keep blood or fluid moving in the right direction.	**Valve**
A qualitative test of blood serum, useful in determining the origin of different types of JAUNDICE and measurements of liver function.	**van den Bergh test**
Chickenpox.	**Varicella**
VARICOSE VEINS.	**Varices**
Varicose, twisted veins of the spermatic cord; a soft mass in the SCROTUM that feels like a bag of worms. The condition occurs most frequently in adolescence and tends to disappear with maturity. Usually it is a minor affliction, often undetected, causing no discomfort, or sometimes a slight dragging feeling, relieved by wearing a suspensory bandage. Varicocele does not significantly affect the health of the testes or lead to impotence or sterility. Only a few cases warrant surgery.	**Varicocele**
Swollen, dilated, tortuous veins. The site most frequently affected is the legs. Varicose veins frequently develop during, or are aggravated by, pregnancy.	**Varicose veins**
Smallpox.	**Variola**
A tube or vessel, usually applied to the vas deferens.	**Vas**
Of or relating to or abundant in vessels, especially blood vessels. Well-vascularized tissues have abundant blood supply; *avascular* tissues such as the CORNEA have none.	**Vascular**
The duct through which SPERMATOZOA are transported from the testicle to the seminal vesicles and urethra.	**Vas deferens**
A simple surgical procedure for sterilization of a man. The excretory duct of the testis (VAS DEFERENS) is severed or a portion cut out of it to prevent SPERMATOZOA from entering the	**Vasectomy**

SEMEN. The structures are close to the surface and the operation can be done under local anaesthesia. There is no interference with sexual capacity since the hormone-producing tissues of the testicle are not affected. It is prudent to regard the sterilization as permanent, although in a few cases the several ends of the ducts have been rejoined, with restoration of fertility. It should be remembered that the sterilizing effect of vasectomy is not immediate. There are still spermatozoa in the seminal vesicles.

Vasoconstrictor

A drug or natural substance or mechanism that narrows the calibre of small blood vessels and reduces the volume of blood flowing through.

Vasodilator

An agent that dilates small blood vessels so that more blood flows through them; blood pressure is usually lowered. The opposite of VASOCONSTRICTOR.

Vasomotor

Of or relating to mechanisms that control dilatation or constriction of walls of blood vessels, and thus the volume of blood flowing through them. Impulses from centres in the brain go to muscle fibres in walls of blood vessels causing constriction or dilatation. Feedback mechanisms of the vasomotor system are exceedingly intricate. In haemorrhage, for instance, the fall in blood pressure caused by loss of blood makes the vasomotor machinery constrict blood vessels and speed the heart, which tends to restore blood pressure to normal.

Vector

A carrier, spreader of disease; especially, an insect or animal host that carries disease germs and transmits them to human beings.

Veins

Thin-walled, strong blood vessels that collect dark used blood from tissues and carry it to the heart at low pressure to be pumped through the lungs, where the blood leaves carbon dioxide and takes up oxygen. Blood from capillaries is collected into *venules* (tiny veins) which enter into larger veins and finally into the *vena cava* which opens into the right atrium of the heart. When a vein is cut the blood wells out in a steady flow with no evident pressure.

CONDYLOMA ACUMINATA.	**Venereal warts**
Bloodletting; same as PHLEBOTOMY.	**Venesection**
A small cavity or chamber; especially, the ventricles of the heart and brain. The lower part of the heart has a right ventricle which receives venous blood and pumps it to the lungs, and a left ventricle which receives oxygenated blood from the lungs and pumps it to the body. The brain has several ventricles filled with CEREBROSPINAL FLUID. Increased volume and pressure of fluid in brain ventricles, due to impaired drainage, results in HYDROCEPHALUS.	**Ventricle**
An X-ray of the brain taken after introducing air or a contrast medium into the ventricles.	**Ventriculogram**
The smallest veins, communicating with capillaries.	**Venules**
Wormshaped.	**Vermiform**
A greasy substance that covers and waterproofs the skin of the fetus.	**Vernix caseosa**
A wart.	**Verruca**
Turning, manipulation of the fetus in the uterus to attain a better delivery, such as turning the feet in podalic version.	**Version**
One of the 33 bones which constitute the spine. Vertebrae are roughly circular bones with knobs for muscle attachments and a hole in the middle for passage of the spinal cord. Individual vertebrae, except those which are fused to form the SACRUM and COCCYX, are separated by pads of elastic cartilage (*intervertebral discs*) which absorb shocks and give a certain amount of flexibility.	**Vertebra** (pl., *vertebrae*)
The highest point of the skull, the topmost part of the head.	**Vertex**
See DIZZINESS.	**Vertigo**

Vesicant	An agent that produces blisters, such as mustard gas.
Vesicle	A small sac containing fluid, like a skin blister.
Viable	Capable of living.
Vibrissae	Hairs in the nose. Also, a cat's whiskers.
Villi	Minute finger-like projections from the surface of a mucous membrane. The small intestine contains millions of villi which increase the surface area in contact with foods.
Vincent's infection	TRENCH MOUTH
Virilism	Development in a female of masculine characteristics (beard growth, deep voice, and so on), usually due to a masculinizing tumour of the ovary, overactivity of the cortex of the adrenal glands, or administration of androgenic hormones.
Viruses	Very small agents that may cause disease.
Visceroptosis	Sagging of abdominal organs from their normal position.
Viscid	Sticky, adhesive.
Viscus (pl., *viscera*)	An internal organ, such as the intestines, stomach, heart, lungs, and kidneys.
Visual field	The area of space seen when the gaze is fixed straight ahead.
Visual purple	A pigment produced by RODS of the RETINA, essential for good vision in dim light. The purplish pigment bleaches to yellow when exposed to light. A product of its breakdown is vitamin A, which is also needed for its regeneration. Severe deficiency of vitamin A causes night blindness because of the inability of visual purple to regenerate adequately.
Vitiligo (*leukoderma*)	Irregular white patches of skin, sometimes streaks of white or grey hair, due to lack of pigment. Often there is a family

tendency to develop the condition. The white patches are most conspicuous when surrounded by deeply tanned skin. No infallible way of inducing repigmentation of the spotty patches is known, but in some instances the taking of an oral drug, *methoxypsoralen*, followed by controlled exposure to sunlight, may produce some deposit of pigment. However, results are uncertain and the treatment may cause some irritation of affected areas and excessive pigmentation of surrounding skin. Vitiligo is not a systemic disease but a purely cosmetic defect which, if distressing, can usually be covered satisfactorily with a tinted preparation.

Transparent colourless material which fills the eyeball behind the lens.	**Vitreous humour**

Twisting or knotting of the bowel, leading to intestinal obstruction and possibly GANGRENE of the part.	**Volvulus**

Forcible ejection of stomach contents. A protective mechanism for getting rid of toxic or irritating materials. Ordinarily, vomiting is a transient event of no great significance in itself, provoked by gastric indiscretion, motion sickness, or some infectious illness accompanied by other symptoms. Vomiting from minor intestinal upsets can be managed simply. Either PROJECTILE VOMITING or COFFEE-GROUND VOMIT is a symptom requiring immediate investigation. Intractable, prolonged vomiting (or diarrhoea) can seriously deplete body fluids and ELECTROLYTES, especially in infants who have small reserves. Common causes of ordinary infant vomiting are stomach dilatation from *overfeeding* (too-frequent feeds or too much at a time) or *underfeeding*, leading to hunger, crying, air-swallowing and distension. Too-hot feeds may induce vomiting. Vomiting may be controlled by ice-cold feeds.	**Vomiting**

GLYCOGEN STORAGE DISEASE with involvement of the heart, liver, and kidneys.	**von Gierke's disease**

See NEUROFIBROMATOSIS.	**von Recklinghausen's disease**

Vulva

The external female sex parts.

Vulvovaginitis

Inflammation of both the VULVA and VAGINA. A severe gonorrhoeal form occasionally is transmitted to female infants and children by careless hygiene. See TRICHOMONIASIS and CANDIDIASIS.

Outward turning of an eye; divergent squint, a condition of ocular muscle imbalance.	**Wall-eye**

Harmless but unsightly small growths from the skin. Common warts of the hands, face, and feet, most fequent in children, are caused by viruses, are contagious, and the sufferer may reinoculate himself over and over again. Common warts can be removed by a great variety of methods, including magic, and they tend to disappear in time with no treatment at all. An isolated wart is probably best left alone, unless it is very disfiguring or painful, or is enlarging or changing its appearance, or is in a part of the body subject to constant irritation. Warts at the edges of fingernails or underneath them are hard to treat; applications of cold – dry ice or liquid nitrogen – are commonly used. Warts in the scalp or beard area are especially troublesome because shaving and combing the hair tend to spread them. A man with warts in the beard area should use an electric shaver. | **Warts** |

The original test for syphilis. It is not specific for syphilis; false positive reactions may be produced by malaria, hepatitis, mononucleosis, and other unrelated diseases. | **Wassermann test** |

HYDROCEPHALUS. | **Water on the brain** |

A method of removing superfluous hair, usually of the legs or lips. A waxy compound is warmed to make it fluid and a layer is applied in the direction in which the hair lies. After the layer has hardened, the sheet is pulled sharply against the direction of hair growth. Embedded hairs are pulled out by the roots. The hair follicle is not permanently destroyed, as it is in ELECTROLYSIS. Fine hair tips reappear in two or three weeks, but wax epilation does not leave a stubble as shaving does. Repeated wax epilation tends to damage some follicles and in time to reduce the number of hairs. Slight irritation lasts for a few hours after wax epilation. The treatment is considered to be safe in competen⁺ hands, but the skin of some women will not tolerate it. | **Wax epilation** |

White blood cell count. | **W.B.C.** |

Weals	Temporary skin swellings resembling mosquito bites, but often much larger. Weals may result from allergy, drugs, irritants, or injection of substances in skin tests of sensitivities.
Webbed fingers	Connection of adjacent fingers by a thin fold of skin between them. A similar condition may affect the toes.
Weber test	A hearing test to determine which ear hears better by bone conduction. It is performed by touching a vibrating tuning fork to various parts of the head.
Weil's disease	An acute feverish illness caused by spirochaetes. A severe form of LEPTOSPIROSIS.
Wen	A sebaceous cyst, a skin tumour ranging up to the size of a marble or larger, filled with cheesy material; movable, firm, rarely painful. Wens usually occur on the scalp, face, or back, and result from obstruction of an oilsecreting gland. They are harmless, and easily removed.
Whiplash injury	A popular term for injury sustained when the head is suddenly thrown forwards and jerked backwards, as in cracking a whip. This may occur in car accidents. The injury is something like a sprained neck; muscles and ligaments may be strained and torn but bones and nerves are rarely damaged.
Whipple's disease	A rare progressive disease of unknown cause characterized by multiple arthritis, fever, fatty stools, lymph node enlargement, diarrhoea, loss of weight and strength, and abnormalities of the small intestine. Antibiotic treatment continued for many months may reverse the course of the disease, which may possibly be of bacterial origin.
Whipworms	Slender worms which inhabit the CAECUM of dogs, pigs, sheep, and goats. Their eggs can be transmitted to man by contact with contaminated soil. The infection may be symptomless or it may produce diarrhoea or acute appendicitis.
Whites	Vaginal discharge; see LEUCORRHOEA.

See PARONYCHIA.

Whitlow

A serious but preventable disease of childhood, especially dangerous and sometimes fatal in young infants whom it readily attacks. It can be prevented by immunization, which is often combined with the toxoids of diptheria and tetanus.

Whooping cough
(*pertussis*)

An ANTIBODY test of blood for the diagnosis of typhoid fever.

Widal test

A malignant tumour of the kidney occurring in children. The tumour may first be noticed as an abdominal mass by mothers in caring for their babies. Early discovery and immediate treatment (surgery and radiation) give the best hope of permanent cure. Simultaneous administration of an antibiotic which causes the tumour to regress has recently been shown to improve the chances of cure.

Wilms tumour

A disease inherited as a recessive trait. Abnormal deposits of copper in many tissues, especially the brain, eyes, kidneys, and liver, cause damage producing various symptoms as the disease progresses: tremor, clumsiness, psychological disturbances, weakness, emaciation, blue half-moons of the nails, retraction of the upper lip exposing the upper teeth. Treatment is directed to decreasing the intake of copper-rich foods (chocolate, molasses, shellfish, kale, liver, peas, nuts, corn, whole-grain cereals, dried beans, mushrooms, lamb, pork, dark meat of chicken), and use of drugs to prevent absorption of copper and speed its excretion.

Wilson's disease
(*hepatolenticular
degeneration*)

A milklike secretion, resembling COLOSTRUM, exuded from the breast of newborn infants of either sex. If left alone, the secretion dwindles and disappears in a few days.

Witch's milk

Physical reactions to withdrawal of certain drugs (narcotics, barbiturates) from persons addicted to them, who have established physical dependence on the drug. The patient has nausea, diarrhoea, a runny nose, watery eyes, chills, waves of gooseflesh. His arms and legs ache, muscles twitch, he perspires and even in hot weather may cover himself with a heavy

Withdrawal symptoms

blanket. Usually the worst is over within a week.

Womb	The UTERUS.
Wood's light	A device used in diagnosing ringworm of the scalp. Light passed through a special glass filter has no visible rays left but the ultraviolet rays are still present, and cause certain fungi to fluoresce.
Wool-sorters' disease	So named because of its occurrence in persons who handle raw animal hides and hairs; *anthrax*.
Wrist drop	Drooping of the hand at the wrist, inability to lift or extend it, due to paralysis or injury of muscles or tendons which extend the fingers and hands.

A form of XANTHOMA occurring as soft yellow-coloured plaques on the eyelids.	**Xanthelasma**
Yellow tumour; a yellowish nodule or slightly raised yellow-coloured patch in the skin.	**Xanthoma**
A generalized condition attended by many deposits of yellowish fatty materials in tissues, due to some disturbance of CHOLESTEROL and LEPID metabolism. A hereditary form characterized by yellowish deposits around tendons, especially in the elbows, wrists, and ankles, may appear early in life. It is transmitted as a dominant trait. In this condition (*familial hypercholesterolaemia*) blood levels of cholesterol are very high and patients have a tendency to develop premature hardening of the arteries. The inborn trait cannot be corrected but blood cholesterol levels may be lowered by stringent dietary restriction of saturated fats.	**Xanthomatosis**
Yellow vision, a condition in which objects look yellow. It sometimes accompanies JAUNDICE.	**Xanthopsia**
Yellow discoloration of the skin, due to eating excessive amounts of carrots and other vegetables which contain pigments (*carotenoids*) that are deposited in the skin. The condition clears up when yellow vegetable intake is restrained. The condition is harmless.	**Xanthosis**
The female sex-determining chromosome: females have two of them, males only one. See CHROMOSOMES. The X chromosome is larger than the Y chromosome and contains some GENES for which there are no complements on the Y chromosome.	**X chromosome**
An epidemic form of encephalitis, first recognized in Australia, now called *Murray Valley encephalitis*.	**X disease**
Dry skin; a mild form of *ichthyosis*. A rare form, *xeroderma pigmentosum*, begins in childhood. Pigmented spots, made worse by sunlight, appear in the skin, and there are scattered TELANGIECTASES.	**Xeroderma**

X

Xerophthalmia

Extreme dryness of membranes which line the eyelids and front of the eye. Lack of tears may cause infection and ulceration of the CORNEA. The condition is associated with NIGHT BLINDNESS and severe deficiency of vitamin A. Specific treatment consists of prescribed daily doses of the vitamin. There are also other causes of xerophthalmia.

Xerostomia

Dryness of the mouth, due to deficient salivary secretion, drugs, dehydration, or secondary to fevers or other diseases.

Xiphoid

Shaped like a sword; applies to the structure at the lower tip of the breastbone.

X-rays (*roentgen rays*)

Electromagnetic radiation of shorter wavelength than visible light. X-rays can penetrate solid substances, produce shadows of structures of different densities on film, and destroy living tissues. Some living cells, said to be RADIOSENSITIVE, are more easily destroyed by X-rays than others; this is the basis for the use of X-rays in the treatment of cancer.

Y

A tropical disease caused by spirochaetes resembling syphilis organisms. It is non-venereal, and possibly transmitted by insect bites. It is characterized by fever, rheumatic pains, red skin eruptions, and destruction of skin and bones of the nose if not treated.

Yaws

The male sex-determining chromosome. See CHROMOSOME.

Y chromosome

An acute, infectious, feverish disease caused by viruses transmitted by the bites of mosquitoes. The disease exists in tropical America where yellow fever is endemic. Travellers should be protected by a vaccine which is highly effective.

Yellow fever

The *macula lutea*, the small spot near the centre of the RETINA which is the focus of finely detailed vision, and coloured vision.

Yellow spot

A milk product formed by the action of acid-producing bacteria. It has the same food value as the milk from which it is made. When made from partially skimmed milk, as it often is, yoghurt is lower in fat, vitamin A, and calories than when it is made from whole milk. Yoghurt is a good source of the other nutrients obtained from milk, especially calcium, riboflavin, and protein.

Yoghurt

Zoonoses	Diseases of animals transmissible to man.
Zoster, zona	SHINGLES.
Zygoma	The cheekbone.
Zygote	The fertilized egg cell before it starts to divide.

Glossary

It is a convenience for doctors to have their own language. *Tonsillectomy* has exactly half the number of syllables of *surgical removal of the tonsils*. Compound words, although apt to be long, convey a great deal of information. Most importantly, as the majority of medical terms are derived from Greek or Latin they form a common language for doctors in different countries. Words such as patella (kneecap), encephalitis (inflammation of the brain), tracheostomy (an artificial opening made into the windpipe), tomography (a special X-ray technique) and countless others would be understood by any doctor speaking a European language, and many speaking other languages. From the building blocks of these basic roots, words can be built up in all sorts of combinations.

a-, an- Absent, lacking, deficient, without. An*aemia*, deficient in blood.

aden- A gland. Ade*noma* is a tumour of glandlike tissue.

alg-, -algia Pain. A prefix such as *neur-* tells where the pain is (*neur*algia).

ambi- Both.

andro- Man, male. An andro*gen* is an agent which produces masculinizing effects.

angi-, angio- Blood or lymph vessel. An angi*oma* is a tumour consisting of blood vessels.

anti- Against. An anti*biotic* is "against life" – in the case of a drug, against the life of disease-causing microbes.

arthro- Joint. Arthro*pathy* is disease affecting a joint.

bleph- Of or relating to the eyelid.

bronch-, broncho- The large air passages.

cardi-, cardio- Of or relating to the heart.

carp- The wrist.

-cele Swelling or herniation of a part, as *hydro*cele, *recto*cele.

-cephal- Of or relating to the head. En*cephal-*, "within the head", pertains to the brain.

cervi- A neck.

chol-, chole- Relating to bile. Chole*sterol* is a substance found in bile.

chon-, chondro- Cartilage.

costo-, costal Of or relating to the ribs.

cranio- Skull. As in cranio*tomy*, incision through a skull bone.

cry-, cryo- Cold.

cyan- Blue.

-cyst- Of or relating to a bladder or sac, normal or abnormal, filled with gas, liquid, or semi-solid material. The root appears in many words concerning the urinary bladder (cyst*ocele*, cyst*itis*).

-cyte, cyto- Cell. *Leuco*cytes are white blood cells.

dent-, dento- Of or relating to a tooth or teeth.

-derm, derma- Skin.

dia- Through.

-dynia Condition of pain, usually with a prefix identifying the affected part.

dys- Difficult, bad. This prefix occurs in large numbers of medical words, since it is attachable to any organ or process that is not functioning well.

-ectomy A cutting out; surgical removal. Denotes any operation in which all or part of a named organ is cut out of the body.

endo- Within, inside, internal. The endo*metrium* is the lining membrane of the uterus.

-enter-, entero- Of or relating to the intestines. *Gastro*enter*itis* is an inflammation of the intestines as well as the stomach.

eryth-, erythro- Redness. An erythro*cyte* is a red blood cell.

eu- Good. A eu*thyroid* person has a thyroid gland that is normal. A eu*phoric* one has a sense of wellbeing.

gastr-, gastro- Of or relating to the stomach.

-gen- Producing, *gen*erating.

glosso- Of or relating to the tongue.

-gogue Eliciting a flow. A *chole*gogue stimulates the flow of bile.

-gram, -graph These roots refer to writing, inscribing. They appear in the names of instruments which record bodily functions on graphs or charts. The *-graph* is the instrument that does the recording; the *-gram* is the record itself, as *electrocardio*graph and *electrocardio*gram.

gyn-, gynae- Woman, female. Gynae*cology* literally means the study and knowledge of woman, but its common meaning is the medical specialty concerned with diseases of women.

haem-, haemato-, -aem- Pertaining to blood. Haema*turia* means blood in the urine. When the roots occur internally in a word, the "h" is often dropped for the sake of pronunciation, leaving *-aem-* to denote blood, as in *anox*aem*ia* (deficiency of oxygen in the blood).

hemi- Half. The prefix is plain enough in hemi*plegia*, half paralysis, affecting one side of the body. It is not so plain in mi*graine* (one-sided headache), a word which shows how language changes through the centuries. The original word was hemi*crania*.

hepar-, hepat- The liver.

hyal- Glassy, transparent.

hyper- Over, above, increased. The usual implication is overactivity or excessive production, as in hyper*thyroidism*.

hypo- Under, below; less, decreased. The two different meanings of this common prefix can be confusing. Hypo*dermic* might mean that a patient has too little skin. The actual meaning is *under* or *beneath* the skin, the proper site for an injection. The majority of "hypo" words, however, denote an insufficiency, lessening, reduction from the norm, as in hypo*glycaemia*, too little sugar in the blood.

hyster-, hystero- Of or relating to the womb.

-ia A suffix indicating "condition", preceded by the name of the affected organ or system, as *pneumon*ia. A doctor wishing to be more specific might call it *pneumonitis*.

-iasis Indicates a condition, as *trichin*iasis.

-iatro- Of or relating to a doctor. A related root, *-iatrist*, denotes a specialist – *psych*iatrist.

idio- One's own, personal, distinct. As in idio*syncrasy*.

inter-   Between.

intra-   Within.

-itis   Inflammation.

labio-   Lips or lip-shaped structures.

leuc-, leuco-   White.

lig-   Binding. A lig*ament* holds two or more bones together.

lipo-   Fat, fatty.

-lith   Stone, calcification. Lith*iasis* is a condition of stone formation.

mamma-, -mast-   Of or relating to the breast. The first root derives from Latin, the second from Greek. *Mamma*- is obvious in *mammal* and *mammary* gland. The *mast*- root is usually limited to terms for diseases, disorders or procedures, as mast*ectomy* (excision of the breast) and mast*oidectomy* (hollowing out of bony processes behind the ear).

mega-, megalo-   Large. The prefix *macro*- has the same meaning.

melan-   Black. The root usually refers in some way to cells that produce *melanin*, the pigment that produces suntan. But it also endures in melan*choly*, "black bile", a gloomy humour once supposed to be the cause of depression.

men-, meno-   Of or relating to menstruation, from the Greek word for "month".

-metr-, metro-   Of or relating to the womb. *Endo*metr*ium* is the lining membrane of the womb.

myelo-   Of or relating to marrow, and also to the spinal cord.

my-, myo-   Of or relating to muscle. My*ocardium* is heart muscle.

necro-   Of or relating to death (of a tissue).

nephr-, nephro-   From the Greek for kidney. See *ren*-.

neur-, neuro-   Of or relating to the nerves.

ocul-, oculo- (Latin) and **ophthalmo-** (Greek)   Both roots refer to the eye, "ophth" words more often to diseases.

odont-, odonto-   Of or relating to a tooth or teeth.

-oid   Like, resembling. *Typh*oid fever resembles typhus fever, or was supposed to when the name was given, but the two diseases are quite different.

olig-, oligo-   Scanty, few, little. Olig*uria* means scanty urine.

-oma   A tumour, not necessarily a malignant one.

onych-, onycho-   Of or relating to the nails of fingers or toes.

oo-   Denotes an egg. Pronounced oh-oh, not ooh. The combining form *oophor-* denotes an ovary.

orchi-   Of or relating to the testicles. Orchi*dectomy* means the removal of a testicle.

ortho-   Straight, correct, normal. Ortho*paedics* literally means straightening out children.

oro-, os-   Mouth, opening, entrance. From the Latin, which also gives *os* another meaning, to complicate matters. See below.

os-, oste-, osteo-   Pertaining to bone. The Latin *os-* is most often associated with anatomical structures, the Greek *osteo-* with conditions involving bone. Osteo*genesis* means formation of bone.

-osis   Indicates a condition of production or increase (*leuco*cy*tosis*, abnormal increase in numbers of white blood cells) or a condition of having parasites or pathogenic agents in the body (*pediculosis*).

-ostomy   Indicates the surgical creation of a mouth, opening, or entrance. The opening may be external, as in *colo*stomy, the creation of an artificial outlet of the colon as a substitute for the anus, or internal, as in *gastroenter*ostomy, establishment of an artificial opening between stomach and intestine. Compare with *-otomy*.

ot-, oto-   Of or relating to the ear. Oto*rrhoea* means a discharge from the ear.

-otomy   Indicates a cutting, a surgical incision (but not the removal of an organ; compare with *-ectomy*). *Myringotomy* means incision of the eardrum.

pachy-   Thick. A pachy*derm* is thick-skinned.

paed-   Child, hence paed*iatrics*.

para- (Greek) Alongside, near, abnormal. As in para*proctitis*, inflammation of tissues near the rectum. A Latin suffix with the same spelling, **-para**, denotes bearing, giving birth, as *multi*para, a woman who has given birth to two or more children.

path-, patho-, -pathy Feeling, suffering, disease. Patho*genic*, producing disease; *entero*pathy, disease of the intestines; patho*logy*, the medical specialty concerned with all aspects of disease. The root appears in the everyday word *sym*pathy (to feel with).

ped- Of or relating to the foot, as in pe*dal*.

-penia Scarcity, deficiency, poverty.

peri- Denoting around, about, surrounding. Peri*odontium* is a word for tissues which surround and support the teeth.

phag-, -phagy Of or relating to eating, ingesting. As in *geo*phagy, dirt eating; *oeso*phagus, the gullet; phago*cyte*, a cell capable of engulfing and ingesting foreign particles.

phleb- Of or relating to a vein. As in phleb*otomy*, cutting into a vein to let blood; phleb*othrombosis*, a condition of clotting in a vein.

plast-, -plasia, -plasty Indicates moulding, formation. An objective of *plastic* surgery, as in *mammo*plasty, an operation for the correction of sagging breasts.

-plegia From a Greek word for stroke; paralysis. *Quadri*plegia means paralysis of all four limbs.

pneumo- (Greek) and **pulmo-** (Latin) Both terms relate to the lungs.

-pnoea Of or relating to breathing. *Dys*pnoea is difficult breathing.

-poiesis Production, formation. *Haemato*poiesis means formation of blood.

poly- Many.

presby- Old. As in presby*opia*, eye changes associated with ageing.

psych-, psycho- Of or relating to the mind, from the Greek word for "soul".

pur-, pus- (Latin) and **pyo-** (Greek) Indicates pus, as in pur*ulent*, *sup*purative, pus*tule*, and pyo*derma*, suppurative disease of the skin.

pyel-, pyelo- Of or relating to the urine-collecting chamber (pelvis) of the kidney.

pyr-, pyret- Indicates fever.

-raphy A suffix indicating a seam, suture, sewing together; usually describes a surgical operation, such as *hernior*raphy, a suture operation for hernia.

ren- Latin for kidney; this root form is usually found in anatomical terms, such as *renal* and *suprarenal*. The Greek-derived root, **nephr-**, usually occurs in words describing diseases, for example, ne*phritis*.

retro- Backward or behind.

-rhag-, -rhagia Indicates a bursting, breaking forth, discharge from a burst vessel; usually denotes bleeding, as in *haemor*rhage, with an aspect of suddenness.

rhin-, rhino- Of or relating to the nose.

-rhoea Indicates a flowing, a discharge, as in *otor*rhoea, discharge from the ear.

scler- Indicating hard, hardness. *Arterio*scle*rosis* is a condition of hardening of the arteries.

somat-, somato- Of or relating to the body.

stom-, stomato- The mouth or a similar opening.

supra- Above, upon.

tachy- Indicates fast, as in tachy*cardia*, abnormally rapid heartbeat.

thromb- Blood clot.

-ur-, ure-, ureo- Of or relating to urine.

urethr-, urethro- Relating to the urethra, the tube leading from the bladder for discharge of urine.

veni-, veno- Relating to the veins.

xanth- Yellow.

xero- Indicates dryness, as xero*stomia*, dryness of the mouth.

Longman Group Limited
Burnt Mill
Harlow
Essex
England

First published 1982
ISBN 582 55546 9

Set in England
by Computer Data Services
Printed in Hong Kong
by Sheck Wah Tong
Printing Press Ltd